NEW ENGLAND INSTITUTE
OF TECHNOLOGY
LEARNING RESOURCES CENTER

AMERICAN ACADEMY OF OTOLARYNGIC ALLERGY
Series Editor
Jacquelynne P. Corey, M.D., F.A.C.S., F.A.A.O.A.

Food Allergy

Edited by

Richard J. Trevino, M.D., F.A.C.S.

Clinical Associate Professor
Department of Otolaryngology
Louisiana State University
Shreveport, Louisiana

Private Practice
San Jose, California

and

Hamilton S. Dixon, M.D.

Assistant Professor
Otolaryngology—Head and Neck Surgery
Vanderbilt University
Nashville, Tennessee

Private Practice
Rome, Georgia

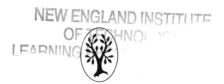

1997
Thieme
New York • Stuttgart

\98

35928137

Thieme New York
381 Park Avenue South
New York, NY 10016

Food Allergy
Richard J. Trevino, M.D., F.A.C.S.
Hamilton S. Dixon, M.D.

Library of Congress Cataloging-in-Publication Data

Food allergy / edited by Richard J. Trevino and Hamilton S. Dixon.
     p. cm.
     Includes bibliographical references and index.
     ISBN 0-86577-618-0. — ISBN 3-13-103721-0 (Stuttgart)
     1. Food allergy. I. Trevino, Richard J. II. Dixon, Hamilton S.
     [DNLM: 1. Food Hypersensitivity. WD 310 F68562 1997]
RC596.F6542   1997
616.97'5—dc21
DNLM/DLC
for Library of Congress   96-49624
                                                                          CIP

Important note: Medical knowledge is ever-changing. As new research and clinical experience broaden our knowledge, changes in treatment and drug therapy may be required. The authors and editors of the material herein have consulted sources believed to be reliable in their efforts to provide information that is complete and in accord with the standards accepted at the time of publication. However, in view of the possibility of human error by the authors, editors, or publisher of the work herein, or changes in medical knowledge, neither the authors, editors, publisher, nor any other party who has been involved in the preparation of this work, warrants that the information contained herein is in every respect accurate or complete, and they are not responsible for any errors or omissions or for the results obtained from use of such information. Readers are encouraged to confirm the information contained herein with other sources. For example, readers are advised to check the product information sheet included in the package of each drug they plan to administer to be certain that the information contained in this publication is accurate and that changes have not been made in the recommended dose or in the contraindications for administration. This recommendation is of particular importance in connection with new or infrequently used drugs.

Some of the product names, patents, and registered designs referred to in this book are in fact registered trademarks or proprietary names even though specific reference to this fact is not always made in the text. Therefore, the appearance of a name without designation as proprietary is not to be construed as a representation by the publisher that it is in the public domain.

Printed in the United States of America

5 4 3 2

TNY ISBN 0-86577-618-0
GTV ISBN 3-13-103721-0

Contents

Contributors

Lynn Danford, M.S.
Department of Otolaryngology
University of Chicago Medical Center
Chicago, Illinois

Hamilton S. Dixon, M.D.
Assistant Professor
Otolaryngology—Head and Neck Surgery
Vanderbilt University
Nashville, Tennessee

Private Practice
Rome, Georgia

Annick M. Gaye, M.D.
Chief of Medical Staff
La Rabida Children's Hospital
Chicago, Illinois

Anil Gungor, M.D.
Clinical Fellow of Rhinology/Allergy
Department of Otolaryngology
University of Chicago Medical Center
Chicago, Illinois

Manisha H. Maskay, Ph.D.
Department of Otolaryngology
University of Chicago Medical Center
Chicago, Illinois

Richard J. Trevino, M.D., F.A.C.S.
Clinical Associate Professor
Department of Otolarnygology
Louisiana State University
Shreveport, Louisiana

Private Practice
San Jose, California

Preface

This is the third volume of the American Academy of Otolaryngic Allergy monograph series on the diagnosis and treatment of allergic conditions. This book deals with immunologically mediated food sensitivities. It will be noted that there are two clinical manifestations of immunologically mediated food sensitivities—the immediate and the more delayed type of sensitivities.

In the first chapter, the immunologic basis of both types of sensitivities will be presented. Following this, IgE-mediated food sensitivities will be discussed by a general allergist. This chapter has been included so that we can be aware of the concepts of IgE-mediated food sensitivities that are espoused by general allergists as well as by otolaryngic allergists. The following chapters will concentrate on non–IgE-mediated food sensitivities and their manifestations, diagnosis, and treatment. A chapter on nutrition rounds out the volume.

I believe that this manual will elucidate immunologically mediated food sensitivities and will give the clinician an immunologic basis for diagnosing and treating this disease complex. This subject matter is still in its developmental phase—as are most known disease complexes—and further study is ongoing and essential for elucidation of all problems and questions arising from food sensitivities.

Food Allergy

◆ 1 ◆

Food Allergies and Hypersensitivities

RICHARD J. TREVINO, M.D., F.A.C.S.

Current data demonstrate that the entire immune system can be activated by foods to produce clinical symptoms. This area of clinical allergy and immunology—the hypersensitivity reactions induced by foods—requires further study. In this chapter, clinical testing and treatment modalities for food allergies will be discussed, as will their immunologic bases described.

The various immune mechanisms involved in the production of tissue damage have been classified into four basic types: I, anaphylactic; II, cytotoxic; III, antigen–antibody complexes; and IV, delayed hypersensitivity.[1] For any immunologic reaction to occur, there must first be penetration of antigenic molecules through a barrier of the body. It has been demonstrated that small, nutritionally insignificant amounts of antigenically intact food macromolecules are transmitted across the mature mammalian gut. For example, insulin injected into an adult rat small intestine has been shown to cause hypoglycemia, suggesting absorption in biologically active quantities.[2] Haptens and larger antigens are absorbed from guinea pig small intestine in quantities that could produce passive cutaneous anaphylaxis.[3] In human subjects, studies have shown that macromolecules, under normal physiologic conditions, can cross the mature mucosal barrier. Fifteen to 30% of normal adults develop milk precipitins after ingestion of milk protein.[4] Earlier studies reported uptake and transport of undigested protein, using a passive cutaneous anaphylactic technique to measure circulating food proteins, and demonstrated precipitins to these proteins in the serum of adults.[5] Thus, food antigens can be absorbed through the gastrointestinal mucosa into the body and stimulate immune responses.

1

The types of immunologic responses incriminated in the production of symptoms caused by food ingestion can be documented.

Type I (Anaphylactic) Reaction

Type I, the anaphylactic reaction, is the classic reaction mediated through IgE, which attaches to the cell membrane of blood basophils or mast cells in the tissues. Vasoactive amines are released from these cells following a reaction between antigen and the antibody IgE. This produces symptoms that may be generalized or localized, depending on the mode and degree of administration of antigen. Generalized anaphylaxis may affect the respiratory tract (bronchial obstruction and laryngeal edema), the gastrointestinal tract (nausea and vomiting, cramping pain, diarrhea, bloating, and occasionally blood in the stool), the cardiovascular system (hypotension and shock), and the skin (hives). Allergic rhinitis and asthma are examples of localized respiratory reactions.

The existence and mechanism of reaginic IgE immediate-onset food sensitivities are well established. Signs and symptoms range from anaphylaxis to urticaria, asthma, rhinitis, vomiting, and diarrhea. The onset is usually within minutes after ingestion and lasts only a few hours. It has been shown that the radioallergosorbent test (RAST) can be used in the diagnosis of food sensitivities. Hoffman and Haddad assembled patients with unequivocal histories of food allergies (ie, ingestion of the food produced a reaction every time it was consumed, and a reaction had occurred within the previous 6 months), often referred to as a fixed food allergy.[6] A number of patients with non–life-threatening symptoms were placed on a strict elimination-challenge regimen to verify the clinical histories. Prick skin testing was performed until two severe systemic reactions resulted in discontinuation of the test. The test group displayed reactions to 14 common foods. Age-matched control sera were tested by RAST and used to determine the normal range for each allergen (Table 1–1).

Table 1–1   Number of Patients with a Positive RAST/Number Tested

FOODS	ANAPHYLAXIS, ANGIOEDEMA, ASTHMA	ECZEMA	URTICARIA SKIN TEST	OTHER SYMPTOMS	CONTROL
Codfish	11/11	5/5	6/7	0/2	0/15
Cow's milk	11/12	15/15	5/5	2/8	0/15
Peanut	3/3	8/8	3/3	0/1	0/15
Orange	5/7	7/9	2/5	0/1	0/15
Egg white	8/9	7/8	9/14	0/2	3/20
Chocolate	7/12	6/10	4/8	0/4	0/20
Walnut	5/5	3/3	6/9	0/1	0/15

Adapted from Hoffman and Haddad.[6]

Allergen systems with adequate allergenic content—that is, more than a contaminant of the extract, such as codfish, peanut, and egg white—produced excellent correlation in patients with severe symptoms; correlation with less defined allergens, such as orange and chocolate, was not significant. Positive RASTs correlate in patients with various symptoms and unequivocal histories (Table 1–2). Note the higher correlation for the more severe symptoms.

These investigators also studied children with severe respiratory allergy without a history of food allergy, finding that 12% were RAST positive to egg. Egg was removed from their diets; this resulted in improvement of the allergic respiratory symptoms; suggesting that some patients previously presumed to have inhalant allergy alone might also have IgE-mediated food allergy. In 1978, May and Brock[7] reported a verification of Hoffman's findings regarding the detection of specific IgE in food-sensitive patients. They found, in a large series, that those who exhibited high serum-specific food IgE levels were sensitive to those foods when challenged orally. There have now been a number of follow-up studies verifying that RAST can be used to diagnose IgE-mediated food sensitivities.[8–17]

Type II and Type III Reactions

Cytotoxic reactions (type II) involve IgG or IgM combining with antigenic determinants on the cell membrane. Alternatively, a free antigen or hapten may be absorbed into the tissue component of the cell membrane, and antibodies subsequently combine with this absorbed antigen. Complement fixation occurs, which often leads to cell damage. The hemolytic reaction induced by a mismatched blood transfusion is a typical example of this type of reaction.

Table 1–2   Correlation of RAST with Symptoms from Food Ingestion in a Group of Patients with Unequivocal Histories

SYMPTOM	NO. OF PATIENTS	% RAST POSITIVE
Anaphylaxis	10	100
Bronchospasm	23	96
Angioedema	13	92
Atopic eczema	30	87
Urticaria	26	62
Diarrhea*	12	92
Acute gastrointestinal upset	6	33
Tension-fatigue syndrome	15	0

*Cases of disaccharidase deficiency, infection, etc, are not included.
Adapted from Hoffman and Haddad.[6]

Type III reactions are caused by the formation of the antigen–antibody complexes circulating in the blood, also utilizing complement. Antigen–antibody complexes form initially, generally in antigen excess, which fix complement. Release of complement components, which are chemotactic for leukocytes, occurs. There is also damage to the platelets, resulting in release of other vasoactive amines. Inflammation and subsequent symptoms result from increased vascular permeability and precipitation of antigen–antibody complexes in capillary walls and tissues. Further fixation of complement and release of chemotactic factors with attraction of polymorphonuclear leukocytes may follow. Neutrophils ingest the immune complexes with release of lysosomal enzymes; this causes further tissue damage and deposition of fibrin. Finally, regression and healing of the lesion may occur if the exposure is a single dose of antigen, or chronic deposition and inflammation will result if there is continuing formation of immune complexes.

Type II or III food sensitivity is much more difficult to diagnose than type I. These reactions are delayed rather than immediate, occurring from 4 hours up to several days after food ingestion. Patients commonly do not relate their symptoms to food ingestion. Investigation of such delayed sensitivities was initiated with the study of complement. In 1936, Lippard et al[18] used complement fixation to detect milk protein and the subsequent appearance of antibody in the serum of infants. Small quantities of milk proteins were found in the first few months of life. The appearance of complement fixation antibodies was followed by the disappearance of antigens from the serum and the presence of precipitating antibodies.

Multiple precipitins to cow's milk have been described, [19,20] as has a change in C3 complement level in a group of young children after oral challenge with a small amount of milk.[21] Some had an immediate reaction and others had a delayed reaction when orally challenged. The group with immediate reaction showed no change in C3, whereas the group with delayed reaction *did* show activation of C3.

In 1977, Sandberg[22] reported a study of children with nephrotic syndrome who had proteinuria after challenge with certain foods. When these foods were withheld from the diet, the nephrotic syndrome cleared and C3 dropped. Sandberg also measured an increase in C3c, an early breakdown product of C3b, indicating that C3 had been activated. He then studied other children, challenging them with various foods, which resulted in a number of delayed symptoms and an elevation of C3c. Sandberg recommended that C3c levels be tested along with any oral challenge test performed.

Although complement change may occur, it is important to remember that C3 can be activated not only by the immune system, but also by the alternative system for complement activation. However, Trevino demonstrated that the delayed food reaction was truly an immunologic reaction.[23] One food showing a positive reaction on the leukocyte-cytotoxic test was chosen for each of 55 patients in the experimental group, and one food that reacted negatively was chosen for each of 10 patients. Each food was withdrawn from the patient's diet for 4 days. The patients were instructed to ingest this food beginning with breakfast on the fifth day. Fifty-three of the 55 patients in the experimental group reported some symptoms ranging from mild irritability, restlessness, and inability to sleep to severe migraine, nausea, vomiting, and angioedema. None of the controls reported symptoms. In those experiencing symptoms, C3 and C4 dropped significantly, with levels returning to normal the day following provocation. The control group evidenced no changes in C3 and C4. C4 activation occurs only by way of the classic pathway (IgG activation); therefore, delayed food hypersensitivity with complement activation is an immunologic phenomenon. Subsequent studies of delayed food sensitivities show that these early components of complements are activated by food antigens. Circulating complement-fixing immune complexes have been found bound to specific food antigen to which patients were clinically sensitive.[24] Such immune complexes were seen in both normal and food-sensitive subjects, but the concentrations were considerably higher and clearance was slower in the food-sensitive patients.

The study of delayed food reactions has progressed from the investigation of complement, showing that complement is activated by way of the classic complement pathway stimulation, to the measurement of immune complexes. More recently, RAST tests for specific food IgG have been developed, and studies continue to document what relationship, if any, exists among high IgG titers, complement use, and production of symptoms.

Type IV Reactions

Cell-mediated immune reactions (type IV) occur as a result of the interaction between actively sensitized lymphocytes and specific antigens. Such reactions are mediated by the release of lymphokines, direct cytotoxicity, or both, occurring without the involvement of antibody or complement. The delayed skin reaction of poison oak—with its characteristic of mononuclear cell infiltrate developing over a period of 24 to 48 hours—is a typical type IV reaction.

Type IV or delayed hypersensitivity food reactions are the most difficult to demonstrate because the T-cell effect develops 24 to even 72 hours after the attachment of antigen to the target cell. The attachment itself may not occur until several hours after ingestion. Garcia et al[25] described an in vitro procedure for T-cell function, the *lymphocyte transformation test* (LTT). When lymphocytes from the blood of sensitized patients are incubated with food antigens, certain foods increase the activity of the lymphocytes, transforming them to a more blastic form, whereas other foods produce no change. May and Alberto[26,27] selected foods positive by the LTT and challenged patients with these foods. After harvesting the lymphocytes, they demonstrated these cells to be active and transformed even when not exposed to in vitro antigen. They postulated that ongoing in vivo proliferation of lymphocytes was induced by antigens absorbed in the challenge procedure. Transformation of lymphocytes not subjected to food antigens in vitro did not occur when the oral challenge was not performed. These studies have been repeated and confirmed by others.[28]

A study of 258 patients with idiopathic chronic urticaria and angioedema was performed using the LTT for foods and additives.[29] The LTT response index was positive in 238 patients: 44 (18.4%) positive to additives, 83 (35.2%) to food extracts, and 111 (46.6%) to both foods and additives. The implicated additives and foods demonstrating a positive LTT response were eliminated from the diets of patients, with complete remission of symptoms in 61.6% partial remission in 22.0% and no change in 16.2%. These investigators concluded that the LTT was accurate in identification of foods responsible for patients' symptoms. Typically, patients with chronic idiopathic urticaria and angioedema have normal levels of total IgE. There is no evidence of IgG-mediated disease; biopsies of lesions demonstrate no vasculitis as observed in immune complex reactions; and there is no necrosis of the vessel walls or presence of nuclear dust. Neutrophils are not prominent in these biopsies, and immunofluorescent studies for the deposition of immunoglobulins and complement are negative. Thus, there is no evidence of a type I IgE-mediated reaction or a type II or III IgE-mediated reaction. Nevertheless, the LTT is positive in these patients; that is, the lymphocytes are stimulated by the foods, and the elimination of these foods improves the condition of the patients.

The immunologic reaction implicated in producing the urticaria is type IV delayed hypersensitivity. In similar experiments involving patients with the allergic tension-fatigue syndrome, total remission occurred in 86.3%.[30] Although these studies do not provide direct evidence of T-cell activity, they do provide deductive evidence. There is more direct evidence from studying enteropathy in patients with food-induced symptoms. Askenazi et al[31] studied cell-mediated immunity within the small intestinal mucosa in celiac disease using a test for T-cell activation by measurement of leukocyte inhibition factor (LIF), which decreases white cell migration. When the patient's T cells and the antigen are incubated together in an agar well, migration from the well (or lack of it) can be easily measured. In a group of patients with celiac disease, this test demonstrated that the disease symptoms resolved when specific foods producing an LIF-positive response were eliminated from the patients' diets. Minor et al[32] measured LIF responses to milk proteins in children with milk-induced enteropathy and verified a positive correlation in 75%. Withdrawal of the milk eliminated the enteropathy. Therefore, T-cell type IV delayed hypersensitivity reactions occur secondary to food antigenic stimulation and cause noxious effects.

All four types of immunologic reactions may be stimulated simultaneously by food antigens, the one causing the most severe symptoms being the one that is recognized.

Food Allergy

Two types of food allergy occur clinically, fixed and cyclic. The response to IgE type I anaphylactic fixed food allergy is usually prompt, seen within minutes to hours. The symptoms produced are the typical anaphylactic reactions, for example, urticaria, wheezing, bronchoconstriction, conjunctivitis, and angioedema. Sensitivity to the food usually persists for more than 2 years after the food is removed from the diet and may last indefinitely. This fixed food allergy is estimated to account for about 5% of all immunologically induced adverse reactions to foods. Therefore, treatment for IgE-mediated food sensitivity is elimination of the offending food.

The second type of food allergy is the cyclic form. This non–IgE-mediated delayed sensitivity accounts for 60 to 80% of the food sensitivity problems seen in clinical practice. These are probably IgG-mediated, representing an immune complex disease. Identification of this type of sensitivity depends primarily on history. Verification may be accomplished with a measurement of specific IgG or immune complexes, but it must be noted that a high level of IgG or immune complexes does not necessarily mean that the person is clinically sensitive to this particular food. The immune response could just be protective in nature. Following the in vitro testing, the foods that show a high IgG level should be tested with an in vivo test.

Cyclic food allergy, unlike fixed food allergy, is exposure-dependent. Increased frequency of ingestion leads to increased sensitivity; that is, the more frequently the food is eaten, the higher the concentration of specific IgG and immune complexes, and the greater probability of symptom production. When exposure is present at nearly every meal, as occurs in such hidden foods as corn or milk, a condition of masked food allergy may occur in which a small amount of the food actually relieves the symptoms for a short period of time. Treatment for this type of food sensitivity is elimination of the food. Elimination need not be indefinite, but rather for 5 to 6 months. The food can then be reintroduced into the diet, but not consumed every day. Foods should be rotated so that exposure to any food is no more frequent than every 4 to 5 days. Infrequent exposure commonly ensures that the specific IgG to these foods will not become elevated and symptom-producing levels will not be reached.

The cyclic pattern of delayed food sensitivity may be explained through an IgG immune complex mechanism (Fig. 1–1). Stage 1 is masked sensitization. The food is eaten frequently, leading to immune complex disease with continuous chronic symptomatology. During this time, there is a phenomenon called *masking* in which a small amount of food is eaten and symptoms are relieved for a short period of time. Masking is explained through the effects of prostaglandin E.

Prostaglandins are intracellular components that function to fine-tune the metabolisms of the cells. Their effect is on the cell itself. They might affect

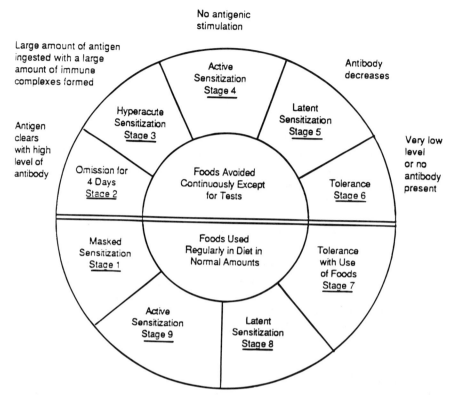

No antigenic
stimulation

Large amount of antigen
ingested with a large
amount of immune
complexes formed

Antibody
decreases

Active
Sensitization
Stage 4

Hyperacute
Sensitization
Stage 3

Latent
Sensitization
Stage 5

Antigen
clears
with high
level of
antibody

Very low
level
or no
antibody
present

Omission for
4 Days
Stage 2

Foods Avoided
Continuously Except
for Tests

Tolerance
Stage 6

Masked
Sensitization
Stage 1

Foods Used
Regularly in Diet in
Normal Amounts

Tolerance
with Use
of Foods
Stage 7

Active
Sensitization
Stage 9

Latent
Sensitization
Stage 8

Figure 1–1.   Increased immune complex disease with increased antigen exposure.
(From Rinkel H.J., Randolph T.G., Zeller M.: Food Allergy. Springfield, IL, Charles
C. Thomas, 1951. Courtesy of Charles C. Thomas, Publisher.)

adjacent cells but have no effect on distant sites, and they are rapidly inactivated in the circulation. There are prostaglandins that have antagonistic actions to each other, but when prostaglandin E predominates, it has an effect on the cyclic nucleotides within the cell. Cyclic AMP is increased and cyclic GMP is decreased intracellularly. This has the effect of making the cell metabolically inactive and resistant to injury. This is the same mechanism utilized by epinephrine to eliminate the effects of anaphylaxis.

Small amounts of a noxious agent cause the cells to produce prostaglandin E. Thus, when a small amount of food is eaten, prostaglandin E is produced and the symptoms of the immune complex disease are alleviated. This effect is transitory, and lasting a few hours. At that time, the effect of the prostaglandins comes to an end and the immune complex symptomatology reasserts itself. Dependence on this masking action for continued well-being often results in food craving or addiction.

If the antigen or the food is omitted for a period of 4 to 5 days (stage 2), the food antigen is cleared from the body; however, a high level of IgG is still being produced. If a large amount of food is then consumed (stage 3), large amounts of immune complexes form and an exacerbation of symptoms occurs. This is the basis of the oral challenge test in which a person acquires exaggerated symptoms after a 4- to 5-day fast from that food.

If the patient continues to omit the food in question from the diet, the level of IgG gradually falls until the tolerance phase is attained (stages 4–6). At this point, there is a very low level of IgG, if any, to that food antigen. If the food is reintroduced, there will be some elevation of IgG; but, with limitation of the exposure interval, the level of IgG needed for symptom production will not be reached (stage 7). In this tolerance phase, the food or foods in question should be rotated and not eaten any more often than every fifth day to prevent symptom recurrence to a particular food. If the allergic individual again ingests the food frequently (stage 8), the immune system will be stimulated to produce IgG, and eventually the immune response will become elevated enough to again produce symptoms (stage 9).

There are several ways to test for food sensitivities. For IgE-mediated allergic reactions, the RAST or other in vitro determination of specific IgE is diagnostic, but rarely necessary, because these food sensitivities are usually well known to the patient, producing immediate reactions. Two types of in vivo testing for the more delayed food sensitivities are available. The oral challenge test involves the elimination of a specific food for a period of 4 to 5 days followed by ingestion of that food in large amounts. If the patient has a delayed IgG type of sensitivity to this food, he or she will respond in an exaggerated symptomatic manner.

There are occasions, however, when certain foods cannot be eliminated or are very difficult to eliminate from the diet, for example, very common foods such as corn, soy, or wheat. Other common foods may be difficult to eliminate for a period of 4 to 5 months and to rotate in the diet, particularly for a person who travels frequently and is dependent on restaurants. In these cases, provocation with neutralization may be utilized.

Neutralization

Three mechanisms (most likely working together) may explain the neutralization phenomenon. Two are immunologic, one is nonimmunologic, and more mechanisms may be involved that are still unknown.

In 1974, Jerne[33] proposed a hypothesis to explain the complex interactions that regulate antibody formation (Fig. 1–2), suggesting that the immune system is self-regulating and is composed of a network of idiotypes and anti-idiotypic antibodies. According to this hypothesis, an antigen elicits the production of an antibody (Ab_1) that creates a unique sequence of amino acids, the idiotype, in its antigen-binding region, distinguishing it from other antibodies. The unique sequence displayed by idiotype 1 (Id_1) may also function as an immunogen in the same host, for this new array of amino acids is not recognized as self and stimulates the production of another

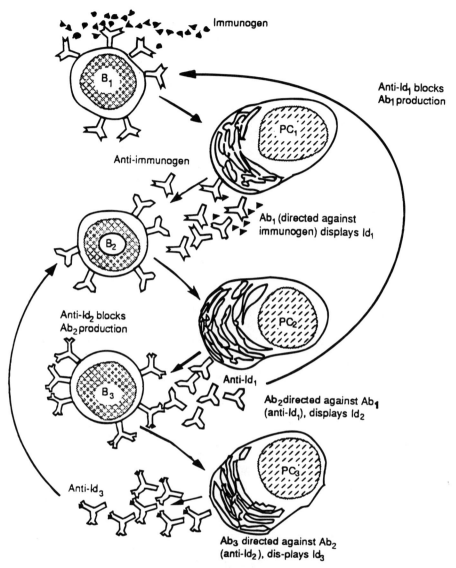

Figure 1–2. Schermatic representation of idiotype—anti-idiotype regulation of antibody formation. (After Jerne.)

antibody (Ab$_2$) that has anti-idiotypic specificity for Ab$_1$. At the same time, it displays another unique idiotype, idiotype 2 (Id$_2$). Ab$_2$ suppresses the production of Ab$_1$. In a similar manner, Ab$_2$ will stimulate the production of Ab$_3$ and its own unique idiotype 3 (Id$_3$), displaying anti-anti-idiotypic antibody against Ab$_2$, and so on, such that each idiotype that is expressed will stimulate the production of a corresponding anti-idiotypic antibody to suppress the production of the antibody (Ab) against which it was produced.

The network can also involve T cells. Helper or suppressor T cells can suppress idiotypes identical to those displayed on antibody molecules. Perturbation of this network initiated by exposure to antigen evolves in interactions between idiotypes, anti-idiotypes, and anti-anti-idiotypes. They either turn on or turn off antibody formation to the activities of the various subsets of immunoregulatory T cells. With low doses of antigen exposure, this regulatory system is shifted toward shutting off Ab_1 to the original immunogen, and the person moves into the low-dose tolerance phase.

The second immunologic mechanism involved with low-dose therapy is the T-cell regulatory system. Proposed cellular interactions that might occur among the already recognized subsets of regulatory T cells are shown schematically in Figure 1–3. This mechanism involves the direct effect of antigen on T cells. Presentation of the immunogen to macrophages results in the activation of helper-effector T cells and helper-suppressor-inducer cells, which cooperate with B cells to initiate antibody formation (pathway 1). At the same time, the helper-suppressor-inducer T-cell population is activated to stimulate the regulator T cells, which influence the suppressor-effector T cells to exert their regulatory suppressor effect (pathway 2).

It is currently believed that the suppressive effects initiated by the suppressor-effector T cells are manifest at the level of the helper-effector T cells rather than by direct action of B cells. In situations in which the immunogen appears to bypass interaction with macrophages (eg, high-antigen dose),

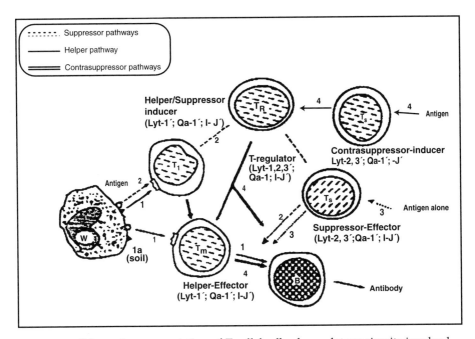

Figure 1–3. Schematic representation of T cell feedback regulatory circuits invalved in the control of antibody formation. (After Gershon and Cantor.)

suppressor-effector T cells can be directly activated by antigen (pathway 3). These cells also exert their suppressive effects at the level of the helper-effector T cell. This pathway may explain the state of pseudotolerance that occurs in the presence of antigen excess.

The final pathway to consider, the contrasuppression circuit (pathway 4), is initiated by the activation of contrasuppressor-inducer T cells. It has a dual regulatory effect, interfering with the suppressive activities of the suppressor-effector T cells as well as rendering the helper-effector T cells resistant to the activity of the suppressor-effector T cell.

With very high antigen stimulation, pathway 3 is dominant, with suppression of antibody production creating the pseudotolerance state. With less antigen administration but still high dose, the level of optimal antibody production is reached and pathway 4 predominates. With less antigen administered or low antigen dose, the suppressive effect through pathway 2 predominates and this is the stage of low-dose tolerance. Thus, with low-dose therapy, the T cell regulatory mechanism shifts more toward the suppression of antibody production. This eliminates immune complex disease.

The third mechanism that protects cells exposed to low-dose antigen exposure is not immunologic but rather involves prostaglandin production. Robert et al[34,35] gave rats oral administration of caustic substances (NaOH, HCl, H_2O_2) inducing extensive necrosis of the gastric mucosa. Pretreatment with exogenous prostaglandin either orally or subcutaneously prevented necrosis. They investigators then produced endogenous prostaglandins by pretreating the rats orally with small amounts of the caustic material. This prevented the necrosis when the caustic concentration of the chemicals was given. They called this phenomenon the cytoprotective effect. Pretreatment of the rats with indomethacin completely ablated the cytoprotective effect of the low-dose oral feeding. Thus, blocking endogenous prostaglandin production blocked the cytoprotective effect.

Based on these findings, Boris et al[36] studied this cytoprotective effect on antigen-induced asthma in humans. In a double-blind study, bronchospasm was evaluated with pulmonary function testing on 19 subjects with a history of wheezing to animal dander. The subjects were challenged with gradually increasing doses of inhaled animal dander until the dose that caused a 20% increase in forced expiratory volume in 1 second (FEV_1) was achieved. Based on intradermal skin end-point titration testing, subjects were pretreated with subcutaneous injection of this end-point dose of animal dander, and the inhalation provocation was repeated. Significant prolongation of the FEV_1 (up to 75%) occurred when an identical inhalation challenge dose was administered. Pretreatment with indomethacin prior to the end-point dose of antigen and rechallenge completely ablated the protection against bronchospasm that was produced by pretreatment with a low dose of injected antigen.

Other studies document antigen-specific desensitization of basophils for high-dose histamine release by low-dose pre-incubation.[37,38] This possible mechanism of neutralization is also supported by a double-blind study of low-dose house dust mite treatment.[39]

Delayed, non IgE mediated food sensitivities may be successfully diagnosed and treated with the application of food antigen on the skin. Mast cell degranulation is effected by many substances other than IgE, including immune complexes and complement (Figure 1-4). Independent documented studies by Breneman, J.C.[40] et al, and Kuwabara, N. et al.[41] confirm that immune complexes together with complement cause mast cell degranulation when food antigens are applied to the dermis. The resulting wheal and flare reaction on the skin is both predictable, and reproducible, making this method of diagnosis and treatment an efficacious option.

This treatment modality, while still in an evolutionary stage of development, may be successfully applied in the diagnosis and treatment of non IgE mediated food sensitivities.

These phenomena have been applied clinically to patients with delayed food sensitivity in a process called *provocation-neutralization.*

The food antigen is first diluted using the standard fivefold dilution method. This is the same process used for preparing inhalant allergies for the serial end-point titration technique.

The dilutions are labeled in numerical order (1,2,3,4,5, etc), with each successive dilution 5 times weaker than the dilution preceding it. Dilution 1 is 5 times weaker than the concentrate; dilution 2 is 5 times weaker than the first dilution, and 25 times weaker than the concentrate, and so on.

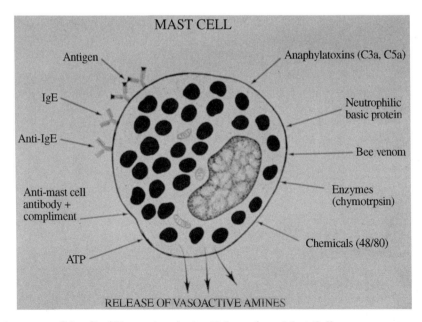

Figure 1–4. Stimuli of Vasoactive Amine Release from Mast Cells.

After intradermal application of 0.05 cm^3 of dilution 1, the skin is observed for a whealing response over a 10-minute period. If there is a progression of swelling before 10 minutes, 0.05 cm^3 of the dilution 2 is applied and observed for 10 minutes. This process of applying successively weaker dilutions continues until a dilution is found which, when applied intradermally, will not provoke a whealing response. This is called the *neutralizing dose,* and it usually occurs at dilution 2 or 3.

This method of testing provides two important pieces of information: it identifies the food to which the patient is reacting, and it identifies the concentration that will provoke prostaglandin E production and "shut off" all the reactive cells.

When possible, this particular food is eliminated from the diet. After 5 to 6 months of elimination, the food can be reintroduced on a rotation basis, every 4 to 5 days.

If the food cannot be eliminated from the diet, the dilution of antigen (determined by testing to be the neutralizing dose) is injected subcutaneously daily, prior to ingestion of the food. This therapy protects the individual from the subsequent ingestion of that food because of the prostaglandin production. After several days of subcutaneous injections of the food antigen, B cells are put into the low-dose tolerant phase. This is due to the B-cell feedback mechanism and the T-cell suppression mechanism, and results in the cessation of IgG formation to that particular food and the subsequent immune complex disease. Continuing antigen therapy over a period of several months results in the progressive diminution of the level of IgG until the patient loses the sensitivity to that food.

The theory and application of low-dose antigen therapy for food sensitivities has been tested in a double-blind fashion by King et al.[42-44] Low-dose therapy gives protection to the shock organ through prostaglandins. The cells of the shock organ, when exposed to a small amount of a noxious substance, produce prostaglandins that cause an increase in cyclic AMP and decrease in cyclic GMP intracellularly, leading to a reduced metabolism and reactivity of the cell. This is the same effect that is produced by the antiasthmatic medication theophylline and the antianaphylactic medication epinephrine. Small doses of immunogen initially protect the cells from the noxious effects of larger doses of the same immunogen. The neutralizing antigen dose is that which causes the shock organ to produce prostaglandins and thus increase cyclic AMP and decreases cyclic GMP, causes the antibody feedback mechanism to shut off antibody production against that antigen, and directly causes suppressor T-cell activity to shut off antibody production. Therefore, small doses of immunogen protect the cells from the damaging effects of larger doses of the same immunogen.

In conclusion, the field of food allergy and sensitivity is a diverse and stimulating one in which food proteins can cause a myriad symptoms via different mechanisms. Clinicians should be aware of all aspects of the immunological response to food sensitivities and be prepared to apply this knowledge in the relief of the patient's symptoms.

References

1. Coombs RR, Gell PG. *Classification of Allergic Reactions Responsible for Clinical Hypersensitivity and Disease: Clinical Aspects of Immunology.* Oxford: Blackwell Scientific Publications;1975:761.
2. Danforth E, Moore RD. Intestinal absorption of insulin in the rat. *Endocrinology* 1959;65:118.
3. Bernstein ID, Ovary Z. Absorption of antigens from the gastrointestinal tract. *Int Arch Allergy Immunol* 1986;33:521.
4. Korenblatt RE, Rothberg RM, Minden P, et al. Immune response of human adults after oral and parenteral exposure to bovine serum albumin. *J Allergy* 1968;41:226.
5. Wilson SJ, Walzer M. Absorption of undigested protein in human being. *Am J Dis Child* 1935;50:49.
6. Hoffman DR, Haddad ZH. Diagnosis of IgE mediated immediate hypersensitivity reaction to foods by radioimmunoassay. *J Allergy Clin Immunol* 1974;54:164.
7. May CD, Brock SA. A modern clinical approach to food hypersensitivity. *Allergy* 1978;33:166.
8. Chua YY, Brenmer K, Lakdawalla N, et al. In vivo and in vitro correlates of food allergy. *J Allergy Clin Immunol* 1976;58:299.
9. Wraith DG, Merrett J, Roth A, et al. Recognition of food-allergic patients and their allergens by the RAST technique and clinical investigation clinic. *Allergy* 1979;9:25.
10. Merrett TG, Merrett J. The RAST principle and the use of mixed allergen: RAST as a screening test for IgE-mediated allergies. *Methods Enzymol* 1980;70:376.
11. Monro J, Brostoff J, Carini C, Zilki K. Food allergy in migraine: study of dietary inclusion and RAST. *Lancet* 1980;2:1.
12. Paganelli R, Levinsky RG. Solid phase radioimmunoassay for detection of circulating food protein antigens in human serum. *J Immunol Methods* 1980;37:333.
13. Schwartz HR, Nerurkar LS, Spies JR, et al. Milk hypersensitivity: RAST studies using new antigens generated by pepsin hydrolysis of beta lacto globulin. *Ann Allergy* 1980;45:242.
14. Freed D. Laboratory diagnosis of food intolerance. *Clin Immunol Allergy* 1982;2:181.
15. Scudamore HH, Philips SF, Swedlund HA, Gleich GJ. Food allergy manifested by eosinophilia, elevated immunoglobulin E level, and protein-losing enteropathy: the syndromes of allergic gastroenteropathy. *J Allergy Clin Immunol* 1982;70:129.
16. Sampson HA, Alberto R. Comparison of results of skin test, RAST, and double-blind, placebo-controlled food challenges in children with atopic dermatitis. *J Allergy Clin Immunol* 1984;6:26.
17. Hattevig G, Kjellman B, Johansson SG, Bjorksten B. Clinical symptoms and IgE responses to common food proteins in atopic and healthy children. *Clin Allergy* 1984;14:551.
18. Lippard VS, Scloss OM, Johnson PA. Immune reactions induced in infants by intestinal absorption of incompletely digested cow's milk protein. *Am J Dis Child* 1936;51:562.
19. Heiner DD, Sears JW, Kniker WT. Multiple precipitins to cow's milk in chronic respiratory disease. *Am J Dis Child* 1962;103:634.
20. Holland HN, Hong R, Davis NC, West CD. Significance of precipitating antibodies to milk proteins in the serum of infants and children. *J Pediatr* 1962;61:181.
21. Mathews TS, Soothill JF. Complement activation after milk feeding in children with cow's milk allergy. *Lancet* 1970;2:893.
22. Sandberg DH, Bernstein CW, McIntosh RM, et al. Severe steroid responsive nephrosis associated with hypersensitivity. *Lancet* 1977;1:388.
23. Trevino RJ. Immunologic mechanisms in the production of food sensitivities. *Laryngoscope* 1982;91:1913.
24. Paganelli R, Levinsky RG, Atherton DJ. Detection of specific antigen within immune complexes: validation of the assay and its application to food antigen-antibody complexes formed in healthy and food allergic subjects. *Clin Exp Immunol* 1981;46:44.
25. Garcia P, Rodriguez JC, Vinos J. A new rapid and more sensitive microcytotoxicity test. *J Immunol Methods* 1971;1:103.
26. May CD, Alberto R. In vitro responses of leukocytes to food proteins in allergic and normal children: lymphocyte stimulation and histamine release. *Clin Allergy* 1972;2:335.
27. May CD, Alberto R. In vivo stimulation of peripheral lymphocytes to proliferation after oral challenge of children allergic to foods. *Int Arch Allergy Immunol* 1972;43:525.
28. Scheinmann P, Gendrel D, Charlas J, et al. Value of lymphoblast transformation test in cow's milk protein intestinal intolerance. *Clin Allergy* 1976;6:515.

29. Valverde E, Vich JM, Garcia-Colderon J, Garcia-Colderon PA. In vitro stimulation of lymphocytes in patients with chronic urticaria induced by additives and foods. *Clin Allergy* 1980;10:691.
30. Valverde E, Vich JM, Garcia-Colderon JV, Garcia-Colderon PA. In vitro response of lymphocytes in patients with allergic tension-fatigue syndrome. *Ann Allergy* 1980;454:185.
31. Askenazi A, Idar O, Handzel ZT, et al. An in vitro immunologic assay for diagnosis of coelic disease. Lancet 1978;1:627.
32. Minor JD, Tolber SG, Frick OL. Leukocyte inhibition factors in delayed onset food allergy. *J Allergy Clin Immunol* 1980;66:319.
33. Jerne NK. Towards a network theory of the immune system. *Ann Immunol* 1974;125c:373.
34. Robert A, Nezamis JE, Lancaster C, Hanchar AJ. Cytoprotection by prostaglandins in rats: prevention of gastric necrosis produced by alcohol, HCl, NaOH, hypertonic NaCCl and thermal injury. *Gastroenterology* 1979;77:761.
35. Robert A. Cytoprotection by prostaglandins. *Gastroenterology* 1979;77:761.
36. Boris M, Schiff M, Weindorf S. Injection of low dose antigen attenuates the response to subsequent bronchoprovocative challenge. *Otolaryngol Head Neck Surg* 1988;98:536.
37. Sobotka AK, Dembo M, Goldstein B, Lichtenstein LM. Antigen specific desensitization of human basophils. *Ann Immunol* 1979;122:511–517.
38. Mendoz GR, Kiminobu M. Subthreshold and suboptimal desensitization of human basophils. *Int Arch Allergy Immunol* 1982;65:101–107.
39. Scadding GK, Brostoff J. Low dose sublingual therapy in patients with allergic rhinitis due to house dust mite. *Clin Allergy* 1986;16:483–491.
40. Breneman JC, et al. Patch Tests Demonstrating Immune Reaction to Foods. *Annals Allergy* 1989;62:461–469.
41. Kuwabara N, et al. Evaluation of patch test with dimethylsulfoxide in association with lymphocyte proliferation in food sensitive atopic dermatitis. *Ped Asthma Allergy & Imm* 1993;7:3 173–178.
42. King W, Rubin W, Fadal R, et al. Provocation-neutralization: a two-part study; Part I: The intracutaneous provocative good test: a multicenter comparison study. *Otolaryngol Head Neck Surg* 1988;99(3):263–271.
43. King W, Fadal R, Ward W, et al. Provocation-neutralization: a two-part study; Part II: Subcutaneous neutralization therapy: a multicenter study. *Otolaryngol Head Neck Surg* 1988;99(3):272–277.
44. King W, Rubin W, Fadal R, et al. Efficacy of alternative tests for delayed-cyclic food hypersensitivity. *Otolaryngol Head Neck Surg* 1989;101(3):385–387.

◆ 2 ◆

Food-Induced Anaphylaxis

ANNICK M. GAYE, M.D., AND ANIL GUNGOR, M.D.

The term *anaphylaxis* was first used at the beginning of the century to describe a fatal reaction upon the injection of a previously tolerated foreign protein, indicating the difference of the event from *prophylaxis*, a beneficial response, commonly obtained by the administration of biologic materials.

Mechanisms

Different mechanisms can trigger this phenomenon (Table 2–1). When foods are implicated in anaphylaxis, the mechanism is usually IgE-mediated. Virtually any food containing proteins can induce the reaction. This reaction can vary from trivial to fatal, progress from local to systemic, involve multiple organ systems, or present as hypovolemic or cardiovascular collapse without warning.

The mediators of anaphylaxis, according to the classical model of mast cell activation by bridging of antigen-specific IgE molecules located on the cell surface, are released in two phases. The preformed granule-associated substances (histamine, enzymes, proteoglycans, and chemotactic factors) are liberated first, followed—4 to 8 hours later—by the newly formed lipid-derived substances (prostaglandins, leukotrienes, and platelet-activating factors) (Table 2–2).

Clinical Manifestations

Anaphylaxis is the clinical expression of the effect of such mediators, massively released, on their target organs. With different degrees of anaphylactic

Table 2–1   Mechanisms of Anaphylaxis

IgE-mediated reactions
Immune complexes/complement
Alteration of arachidonic acid metabolism
Direct mast cell degranulation
Physical
Idiopathic

severity, the skin will present urticaria and angioedema; the respiratory tree, laryngeal edema and bronchospasm; the gastrointestinal tract, nausea, vomiting, and diarrhea; the cardiovascular system, hypotension and dysrhythmia; and the patient will overall have an intense feeling of impending doom, with diaphoresis, palm and groin pruritus, and headache or faintness. Milder reactions may cause only profuse epiphora, rhinorrhea, and drooling with cutaneous tingling and anxiety. The clinical manifestations usually follow closely the exposure to the offending food but may be delayed by the intake of medications or other aliments slowing down the digestion of the meal.

In exercise-induced food-related anaphylaxis, the ingestion of a specific food is essential to the development of the reaction in some patients and appears to only promote or enhance the reaction in others. The occurrence of the reaction is not related to the intensity of the exercise.[1]

Biphasic anaphylaxis has been reported.[2] This presentation could correspond to the late phase of the IgE-mediated reaction, involving the newly formed mediators discussed above, or the expression of a partially treated anaphylaxis episode. The possibility of a late-phase etiology has serious implications in the treatment of the acute anaphylaxis presentation in terms of medications and duration of medical observation. Protracted anaphylaxis is seen when vasopressors do not reverse the cardiovascular symptoms.[2,3] This is most often observed when the patient happens to be taking beta-adrenergic blockers.[4,5]

Table 2–2   Mediators of Anaphylaxis

MEDIATOR	ACTION(S)	SIGNS/SYMPTOMS
Histamine	Vasodilatation	Pruritus, swelling, hypotension, diarrhea
	Bronchoconstriction	Wheezing
Leukotrienes (C_4, D_4)	Bronchoconstriction	Wheezing
	Vasodilatation	Swelling
Platelet-activating factors	Bronchoconstriction	Wheezing
	Vasodilatation	Hypotension
C3a, C5a	Smooth muscle contraction	Wheezing
	Vasodilatation	Hypotension

Table 2–3 Differential Diagnosis

	SIMILARITIES WITH ANAPHYLAXIS	DIFFERENTIATING FEATURES FROM ANAPHYLAXIS
Vasovagal syncope	Pallor, sweating Faintness Nausea	Absence of respiratory symptoms Bradycardia No pruritus, urticaria, angioedema
Hyperventilation	Sweating Aching limbs Nausea Tachycardia Tingling, paresthesia	Maintenance of blood pressure Absence of wheezing and stridor No pruritus, urticaria, angioedema
Globus hystericus	Sensation of upper respiratory obstruction	Absence of wheezing and stridor No evidence of anatomical obstruction Chronicity of sensation No pruritus, urticaria, angioedema No gastrointestinal symptoms Maintenance of blood pressure
Angioneurotic edema	Upper respiratory obstruction Abdominal cramps Angioedema No family history in *acquired* C_1 esterase inhibitor deficiency	No pruritus, urticaria No vascular collapse Slow progression Family history and/or personal history of attacks in *familial* C_1 esterase inhibitor deficiency or dysfunction Low C4 during attacks C_1 esterase inhibitor low or dysfunctional
Serum sickness	Urticaria, angioedema	No pruritus No respiratory obstruction No vascular collapse Fever, arthralgia Purpura
Cold-induced urticaria	Urticaria, angioedema Respiratory obstruction Vascular collapse	Evidence of sudden and strong generalized cold stimulus
Carcinoid syndrome	Gastrointestinal symptoms Flushing Bronchospasm	Increased level of urinary 5-HIAA No urticaria, angioedema No upper respiratory obstruction Recurrence

Table 2–3   Continued

	SIMILARITIES WITH ANAPHYLAXIS	DIFFERENTIATING FEATURES FROM ANAPHYLAXIS
Systemic mastocytosis	Flushing, urticaria Gastrointestinal symptoms Bronchospasm (although infrequent) Increased level of histamine and tryptase	No upper respiratory obstruction Recurrence of attacks with baseline symptomatology Skin lesions with Darier's sign

Although the real incidence of food-induced anaphylaxis is unknown, its fatality rate has been estimated to be higher than that of insect stings.[6] Upper and lower airway obstruction accounts for most (70%) fatalities and cardiovascular events, secondary to hypovolemic shock for most of the remainder of the deaths. Mortality usually occurs early in the clinical syndrome, but significant morbidity, secondary to hypoperfusion of vital organs, may lead to delayed demise.[7] Pathologic examination may reveal laryngeal edema and pulmonary hyperinflation, edema, hemorrhage, and atelectasis. Visceral congestion and myocardial necrosis have also been reported.

Diagnosis

The diagnosis of systemic anaphylaxis is usually readily evident. Most of the multiple causes of respiratory obstruction and vascular collapse can be quickly excluded. Some disease entities present striking similarities with anaphylaxis and deserve closer attention (Table 2–3).

The laboratory evaluation of the patient in anaphylaxis will reveal the different organs affected by the hypovolemic shock. To document the etiology, an elevated serum level of histamine would be most relevant, but this elevation is brief and peaks within 30 minutes of mast cell degranulation. Its measurement is, therefore, not helpful. Another marker of mast cell activation is the elevation of serum tryptase, whose level is sustained for 4–6 hours after antigen challenge, peaking 1 to 2 hours after the onset of anaphylaxis.[8–10]

After the anaphylactic episode, a diagnostic evaluation—including history, detection of food-specific IgE, and, as necessary, careful challenge under supervision—should be undertaken until the offending food allergen is identified.

Treatment

Strict adherence to a scrupulous avoidance diet is essential in this life-threatening syndrome. This must be strongly stressed to patients. Such patients should be taught how to use, and carry on their person, an auto-injectable dose of adrenaline along with precalculated doses of liquid

Table 2–4   Schematic Anaphylactic Shock Management

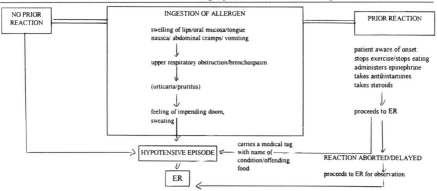

1. SUBCUTANEOUS EPINEPHRINE—may be repeated every 15–20 minutes
   adult: 0.3–0.5 cm^3 (1/1.000)
   child: 0.01 cm^3/kg max 0.5 cm^3 (1/1000)

2. AIRWAY MAINTENANCE
   upper: intratracheal or nasotracheal tube placement tracheostomy as required
   lower: beta-adrenergic nebulization theophylline bolus 5 mg/kg IV/20 min
      then drip
   oxygen by mask or cannula

3. CARDIOVASCULAR MAINTENANCE
   • intravenous/intramuscular diphenhydramine 50–100 mg
   • intravenous line for pressure maintenance
   —fluids
   —alpha agonist as necessary (dopamine, isoproterenol)
   • H2 antagonists
   • glucagon if history of beta blockers
   • MAST (military anti-shock trousers)

4. PREVENTION of late-phase reaction
   hydrocortisone 100 mg IV q 6–8 hrs
   or methylprednisolone 40 mg IV q 6–8 hrs

5. OBSERVATION
6. EDUCATION prior to discharge: avoidance/medications/symptoms
7. FOLLOW-UP
   • identification of allergen
   • education
   • dietitian's input as necessary

antihistamines (H_1 antagonist) and steroids. A medical identification bracelet or necklace is strongly recommended.

The physician should review with patients the circumstances most often associated with fatal outcome to heighten their awareness of these situations where death can be prevented:

- Failure to inquire about the ingredients in a meal prepared by a person not apprised of the possibility of a reaction
- Failure to appreciate the onset of a reaction
  failure to administer epinephrine
  reliance on oral antihistamine alone
- Concomitant intake of alcohol
- Exercise within 6 hours of food ingestion in case of exercise-induced food-associated anaphylaxis
- Use of beta blockers

The dietitian or nutritionist will then educate the patients further about possible cross-reacting allergens, interpretation of food labels, and necessary aliment substitution for a well-balanced diet.

Treatment of Acute Anaphylaxis

Immediate medical attention is most important. Preservation of the airway and maintenance of blood pressure are the two critical issues (Table 2–4).

References

1. Dohi M, Suko M, Sugiyama H, et al. Food-dependent, exercise-induced anaphylaxis: a study of 11 Japanese cases. *J Allergy Clin Immunol* 1991;87:37–40.
2. Stark BJ, Sullivan TJ. Biphasic and protracted anaphylaxis. *J Allergy Clin Immunol* 1986;78:76–83.
3. Sampson HA, Mendelson L, Rosen JP. Fatal and near-fatal anaphylactic reactions to food in children and adolescents. *N Engl J Med* 1992;327:380–384.
4. Marquardt DL, Wasserman SI. Anaphylaxis. In Middleton, ed. *Allergy,* 4th ed. St Louis: Mosby Year Book; 1993;1525–1536.
5. Toogood JH. Risk of anaphylaxis in patients receiving beta-blocker drugs. *J Allergy Clin Immunol* 1988;81:1–5.
6. Yuninger JW. Lethal food allergy in children. *N Engl J Med* 1992;327:421–422.
7. Barnard JH. Studies of 400 Hymenoptera sting deaths in the United States. *J Allergy Clin Immunol* 1973;52:259.
8. Schwartz LB, Yuninger JW, Miller J, et al. Time course and appearance and disappearance of human mast cell tryptase in the circulation after anaphylaxis. *J Clin Immunol* 1989;83:1551.
9. Schwartz LB, Metcalfe DD, Miller JS, et al. Tryptase levels as an indicator of mast cell activation in systematic anaphylaxis and mastocystosis. *N Engl J Med* 1987;316:1622.
10. Smith PL, Kagey-Sobotka A, Bleecker ER, et al. Physiologic manifestations of human anaphylaxis. *J Clin Invest* 1980;66:1072–1080.

◆ 3 ◆

IgE-Mediated Food Allergy

ANNICK M. GAYE, M.D., AND ANIL GUNGOR, M.D.

The label *food allergy* has been applied to a multitude of unexpected clinical manifestations occurring after an encounter with products that our species places in the category of foodstuffs. However, in the medical literature the use of the term *allergy* implies an immunologically related, IgE- or non–IgE-mediated, mechanism of disease.[1] Such a mechanism, after ingestion of a specific food, seems to occur with a prevalence of only 1 or 2% in the adult population and up to 3% in the pediatric age group. Therefore, the term *adverse reaction* is more appropriate to describe any ill presentation after a specific food exposure. Adverse reactions are estimated to occur in up to 33% of adults and 8% of children.[2] The classification of the adverse reactions to food was initiated in 1984 by the American Academy of Allergy and Immunology and the National Institute for Allergy and Infections Diseases[3] and updated in 1994 by the European Academy of Allergy and Clinical Immunology[4] (Tables 3–1 through 3–4).

Clinical Presentations

The atopic syndrome, clinical expression of the genetic predisposition to develop immediate or IgE-mediated allergic reactions, can present in various ways. Atopic dermatitis, asthma, allergic rhino-conjunctivitis, and IgE-mediated food allergies,—the various facets of this syndrome—present simultaneously at different degrees of severity or in a continuum with respective age-related peaks of severity in an affected individual. The peak prevalence of food allergies is around the first year of life. This prevalence decreases to adult levels by the child's fourth birthday.

Table 3–1   Prevalence of Food-induced Reactions

	ADVERSE	IgE-MEDIATED
Adults	33%	1–2%
Children	8%	3%

Atopic dermatitis usually presents in the first 2 years of life (infantile eczema), with a wide spectrum of severity. The patients who are most affected usually have a high total serum IgE level on exposure to common inhalants and occasionally to foods. However, because only 80% of patients with atopic dermatitis have elevated IgE levels and positive skin tests, the role of the IgE-mediated mechanism in the etiology of this disorder is not as clear as in the other manifestations of the atopic syndrome. The most common allergenic foods in infants with atopic dermatitis are cow's milk, fish, and eggs.[5,6]

About one third of patients with atopic dermatitis, especially children,[7] have IgE-triggered cutaneous symptoms to common foods; some describe also late-occurring symptoms of pruritus up to 24 hours after the noxious encounter. Occasionally, the skin manifestations clearly mimic the late phase of the IgE-mediated reaction, now considered to be the cause of airway hyperresponsiveness in asthma. In these cases, the dermatitis pattern will closely follow the distribution of the acute cutaneous reaction.

Mechanisms that are unrelated to IgE-mediated histamine release, but nevertheless trigger mast cell degranulation, may exacerbate atopic dermatitis after the ingestion of alcohol, spicy foods, or additives.

IgE-mediated asthma or reversible obstructive airway disease can be exacerbated by the inhalation of airborne proteins of an offending food such as fish being prepared for a meal or, more chronically and on a larger scale, in the food processing industry[8] (Table 3–5). Food-related asthma can also be triggered by the ingestion route,[9] especially in children, in whom the hyperresponsiveness of the airway condition may be heightened by the repeated exposure

Table 3–2   Adverse Reactions to Food

Toxic (see Table 3–3)

Nontoxic
  Immune-mediated: Food allergy
    IgE (including anaphylaxis)
    Non-IgE (including anaphylactoid reaction)

  Non–immune-mediated: Food intolerance
    Enzymatic or/and metabolic (see Table 3–3)
    Pharmacological (see Table 3–3)
    Psychological (see Table 3–4)
    Undefined

Table 3–3 Some Causes of Non–Immune Mediated Adverse Food Reactions

	FOODSTUFF	CAUSE
Toxic	Shellfish	Saxitoxin
	Grouper, snapper, barracuda	Ciguatera poisoning
	Tuna, mackerel	Scombroid poisoning
	Canned foods	Clostridium botulinum
	Manually prepared meals	*Staphylococcus aureus*
	Cereals	Ergot
	Peanuts	Aflatoxin
	Lima beans, millet sprouts	Cyanogenic glycosides
Pharmacologic	Coffee, colas	Caffeine, methylxantines
	Banana	Serotonin, theobromine, methylxantines
	Chocolate	Phenylethylamine, theobromine
	Tea	Methylxantines, theobromine
	Tomato	Tryptamine, serotonin
	Potato	Glycoalkaloids
	Plum	Tryptamine
	Fish	Histamine, histidine
	Sauerkraut	Histamine
	Cheeses	Tyramine, histamine
	Pickled herring	Tyramine
	Certain mushrooms	Disulfiram-like agent
	Pineapple	Vasoactive amines
	Licorice	Mineralocorticoid-like agent
Enzymatic		Congenital or acquired deficiency of:
	Phenylalanine-containing food	Phenylalanine hydroxylase
	Fructose	Fructose-1-phoshate-aldolase
	Galactose	Galactose-1-phosphate-uridyl transferase
	Lactose	Lactase
	Alcohol	Aldehyde dehydrogenase
	Glucose; lactose; galactose	Cellular transport level abnormality
	Fava beans (ingestion or pollen inhalation)	Glucose-6-phosphate dehydrogenase

to common allergens. Isolated food-induced wheezing is rare: most children have a history of atopic dermatitis or present with the actual skin disorder.[10]

Sodium metabisulfite, a preservative, causes bronchoconstriction in susceptible asthmatics via inhalation of the irritant sulfites released after ingestion. This phenomenon is not immunologically mediated.

Hypersensitivity pneumonitis or extrinsic allergic alveolitis, most often occurring in non-atopic patients, is immunologically mediated. Its triggers,

Table 3–4 Food Aversion or Hyperventilation Syndrome

Triggers	Smell, sight, (auto) suggestion ingestion of a specific food
Presentation	Nausea, weakness, sweating, lightheadedness, aches, tingling, fainting spell
Course	Variable
Investigation	Symptoms reproducible after 1–3 minutes of forced hyperventilation or open challenge but not after blind challenge

Table 3–5 Foods Implicated in Occupational Asthma

Egg
Grain flour: wheat, rye, oat, barley, buckwheat
Coffee bean (green)
Cocoa
Peanut
Soy
Cottonseed
Sunflower
Garlic
Tea
Papaya (papain)
Pineapple (bromelin)
Poultry, pig, cow, rabbit
Fish
Crab, shrimp, prawn, sea-squirt
Hops
Vegetable gum (tragacanth, karaya)

also well known in the food industry, induce an IgM and IgG response and a characteristic symptom complex[11] (Table 3–6).

Urticaria, a pruritic wheal-and-flare cutaneous eruption, presents with macular or annular lesions, isolated or coalescing as they evolve. Each lesion usually lasts less than 24 hours. By definition, acute urticaria is less than 12 weeks in duration.

Table 3–6 Food-Related Occupational Hypersensitivity Pneumonitis

OCCUPATION	FOOD	AGENT
Malt worker	Barley	*Aspergillus clavatus*
Cheese washer	Cheeses	Penicillin species
Poultry handler/feather plucker	Turkey/chicken/duck	Bird proteins
Paprika splitter	Paprika dust	*Mucor stolonifer*
Mushroom worker	Compost	Thermophilic actinomycetes
Honey processor/beekeeper	Honey	Honeybee body parts
Sugarcane handler	Pressed sugarcane (bagasse)	Thermophilic actinomycetes

Angioedema is manifested by areas of cutaneous or mucosal nonpruritic swelling, developing suddenly and lasting no more than 3 days. Urticaria is present in association with angioedema in more than 45% of the cases. When urticaria and angioedema are so extensive and so severe that systemic symptoms are present, such as headache, cough, hoarseness, wheezing, vomiting, abdominal pain, diarrhea, dizziness, and syncope, the term *anaphylaxis* is appropriate. Regardless of its etiology—IgE-mediated, acute allergic or non-immunologically related, pseudo-allergic—urticaria may lead to hypovolemic collapse in a few minutes to half an hour. In the majority of the cases of urticaria and angioedema, no underlying cause can be identified. IgE-mediated urticaria to ingested food represents up to 5% of acute allergic urticaria presenting to the dermatologist.[12]

Pseudo-allergic reactions may occur on first exposure, they are not substance-specific, but they are dose related. A disruption of the arachidonic acid metabolism (eg, by salicylate ingestion) or a direct mast cell release of histamine (eg, triggered by poppy seeds) are the two most obvious causes known of this phenomenon (Table 3–7). When the urticaria or the angioedema has been present daily or repeatedly for longer than 6–12 weeks, the condition is termed chronic, and most often is not an immunologically mediated mechanism. Some food additives may play a role in a few patients. An identifiable food allergy can be found in only 5 or 10% of the patients with chronic urticaria and angioedema.

IgE-mediated urticaria upon cutaneous contact[13] with food may occur after respiratory, gastrointestinal, or dermatologic sensitization. This contact usually happens during the preparation of a meal when the food is raw and handled for long periods, such as in kneading, cutting, or paring (Table 3–8).

Table 3–7   Foods Implicated in Urticaria-Angioedema

ACUTE ALLERGIC	PSEUDO-ALLERGIC
	Dyes:
Fish	Tartrazine (orange)
Shellfish	Sunset yellow
Milk	Ponceau (red)
Nuts	Erythrosine (red)
Beans	Amaranta (red)
Potatoes	Indigotine (blue)
Celery	Brilliant blue
Parsley	Preservatives:
Spices	Benzoic acid
Peanuts	Salicylates
Soy	Parabens
	Sulfites
	Antioxidants
	Ascorbic acid

Table 3–8   Foods Implicated in Contact Urticaria

Egg (white)
Seafood
Wheat, rye, malt flour and dough
Chicken, turkey
Lamb, beef
Potato
Carrot, celery, apple, banana, lettuce, endive, garlic
Milk
Spices

The *oral allergy syndrome (OAS)* is one of the most common forms of IgE-mediated food allergy in adults.[14,15] Although it is recognized that food-related IgE reactions may occur minutes to hours after ingestion, in OAS the correlation between the offending food and the immediacy of the local reaction is readily made by the patients, who therefore may never seek medical attention. Immediate swelling of the lips, tingling of the tongue and throat and blistering of the oral mucosa are easily recognized and are enough of a warning. The oral allergy syndrome occurs in up to 40% of patients with pollenosis when they are exposed to fresh fruits and vegetables that cross-react with their specific allergic rhinitis–inducing pollen[16] (Table 3–9).

The *gastrointestinal anaphylactic syndrome,* IgE-mediated, is the localized expression of a reaction usually occurring systemically: it is rarely seen without other manifestations of immediate allergy such as urticaria or respiratory problems. Nausea, vomiting, abdominal cramps, and diarrhea are common, immediate, and severe.

In *IgE-mediated eosinophilic gastroenteritis,* patients, usually atopic, have an elevated IgE level and peripheral eosinophil count and many significant skin tests to foods and inhalants. The features of pyloric obstruction with early satiety, postprandial nausea, emesis, and weight loss or failure to thrive are elucidated when, upon endoscopic biopsy, diffuse eosinophilic infiltration of the gastric outlet is demonstrated; this occasionally extends throughout the gastrointestinal tract. Strict avoidance of the offending foods brings relief of symptoms. Another group of patients with similar symptoms

Table 3–9   Oral Allergy Syndrome: Cross-Reactivity Between Aeroallergen and Food Components

INHALANT	FOOD
Ragweed	Melon, watermelon, gourds, banana
Birch	Apple, carrot, potato, celery, fennel, kiwi, hazelnut, pear, peach
Mugwort	Celery
Grass	Tomato, melon, watermelon, kiwi
Hazel	Hazelnut
Unknown	Cherry, plum, apricot, peach
Dust mite	Snail, shrimp

and eosinophilic gastrointestinal dissemination, although seemingly non-atopic, may respond to the introduction of an elemental diet.[17]

Infantile colics, in about 15% of the children affected, seem secondary to IgE-mediated food allergy.[18]

Pathogenesis

Any food can be allergenic. Made of fat, carbohydrates, and proteins, each food can have more than a single antigenic component. These components are usually water-soluble glycoproteins,[19-21] with a molecular weight of 10–60 kDa. These glycoproteins are most often heat, acid, and enzyme stable, resisting home or factory processing, gastric acid degradation, and intestinal enzymatic metabolism. The major food allergens in children are egg white, cow's milk, peanuts, soy, fish, and wheat. In adults nuts, peanuts, fish, and shellfish account for most reactions.[22] The causative foods have a different distribution throughout the world, representing the different ethnic preferences and agricultural availabilities. For instance, rice allergy is more prevalent in Asia, peanut sensitivity more so in the United States.

Cross-allergenicity among related members of food families was long thought to occur; it is commonly observed by skin or in vitro testing but is no longer considered clinically relevant.[23] Large studies have shown that among food-allergic children, less than 1% have hypersensitivity to more than one member of a food family and that only 11% are allergic to more than one food, more commonly peanut and egg or milk and egg.[24] When counseling patients with legume[25,26] (eg, peanut), cereal[27] (eg, wheat), or "dairy" (eg, milk or egg[24]) products sensitivity, overly restrictive diet involving the complete family of foods is not scientifically warranted or nutritionally appropriate. In contrast, adequate studies of the shellfish (crustaceans and mollusks) and the nut families have not been done yet.[23] The sensitivity to shellfish[28] and tree nut is usually severe and permanent. A diet that restricts these food groups is not nutritionally compromising.

Patients allergic to fish, however, are very often sensitive to multiple fish species[29,30] and, if the consumption of fish is deemed culturally or nutritionally necessary, specific challenge in a controlled setting should be done before recommending any particular regimen.[23]

The allergens specifically responsible for the oral allergy syndrome are often very labile to heat and processing, and seem to be of two categories:[31] (1) primary allergens, causing generalized clinical symptoms, and (2) secondary allergens, divided between profilins, present in distantly or unrelated plants and food groups, and cross-reacting carbohydrate determinants, present in most vegetables and invertebrates. The symptoms are more severe during the pollen season of the plant (eg, birch), when the pollen-allergic patient eats the raw cross-reacting food (eg, apple or hazelnut).[15,32] The contact of the intact secondary allergens with the oral mucosa mast cells is apparently a necessary trigger for the reaction.

Small and large molecular weight chemicals naturally occurring in food or used in processing may cause IgE-mediated reactions. Some of these allergens occur in gelatin, vegetable gums, formalin, and ethylene oxide.[33]

Other mechanisms, non-immunologically related, account for the low molecular weight substances causing other adverse reactions: vasodilatation (eg, sodium nitrite) or irritation (eg, monosodium glutamate in high concentration).

Diagnostic Evaluation

Despite the notorious unreliability of most patients' memory in regard to their food intake, obtaining a detailed sequence of events with an evaluation of the amount of food ingested, timing of symptoms, and their description is most helpful as the first diagnostic step of IgE-mediated food allergy: a food diary. After one obtains a complete medical history and the results of skin tests and radioallergosorbent test (RAST), an elimination diet[34] removing all foods to which the patient had specific IgE antibodies is then undertaken. In IgE-mediated food problems, 2 weeks of this diet should bring about almost complete resolution of the symptoms. Challenges with one suspected food at a time—open, single-blinded, double-blinded, placebo-controlled if necessary—will then confirm or rule out the need for a restrictive diet.[35] Even a negative carefully designed placebo-controlled food challenge does not rule out the possibility of an IgE-mediated reaction. Indeed, some patients may remain asymptomatic until the offending food is given on repeated occasions or in large amounts. In other rare circumstances, the food-induced reaction may need a sine qua non trigger like physical exercise to express itself.[36] The symptom severity, related by history, will guide the choice of setting for these challenges. All negative blind challenges must be confirmed by an open feeding challenge under observation. A standardized scoring system is then used to assess the reactions.[35] Rechallenges are usually recommended every 2–3 years of a specific restrictive diet, except for foods such as fish, shellfish, nuts, and peanuts, whose effects should be considered permanent.

Traditionally the most used method of testing, the food prick test nevertheless lacks at this time the extract standardization physicians have learned to trust in the diagnosis of inhaled allergies. The development of standardized allergenic extracts depends on the identification of the major allergens in specific foods. Considerable work has recognized over 20 protein fractions in cow's milk; four major egg white allergens; two peanut, two soybean, one codfish, and six shrimp allergens.[23] The translation of these well-defined food allergens into extracts of clinical relevance is under way. At this time, however, well performed skin tests are greater than 95% accurate for ruling out IgE-mediated food allergy, but 70% to not at all helpful in diagnosing it.[37] IgE RAST does not significantly change these predictive odds.[38] Studies have been undertaken to increase the accuracy of in vitro testing by other methods. The in vitro methods are the tools of choice in anaphylactically sensitive patients, in repeatedly severe skin reactions, or when antihistamines are taken to control an associated chronic condition.

When all tests are inconclusive, and the suspicion of an IgE-mediated reaction remains high, an intragastric provocation under endoscopic control, followed by biopsy, can be considered and has been infrequently used.[39]

Other tests including food-specific IgG, IgA, and IgM levels will indicate exposure rather than sensitivity to these foods.[40] Studies of absorption or digestion (D-xylose, vitamin levels, stool for fat, blood, eosinophils) are more valuable in non–IgE-mediated gastroenteropathy management.[40]

Treatment

Once immediate IgE-mediated allergy is demonstrated, the only logical and proven mode of therapy is to avoid the offending allergen. When a major food needs to be eliminated, the alimentary regime may become nutritionally hazardous. A dietitian's advice is most helpful with the calculation of appropriate protein substitution and mineral and vitamin supplements, especially for growing children and pregnant women.[41]

Up to a third of children allergic to cow's milk protein will develop soy sensitivity; this is especially true for non–IgE-mediated milk-induced syndrome.

Loss of clinical sensitivity to the implicated food allergens occurs over time on a restrictive diet, most often with soy and less frequently with wheat, egg, and cow's milk. The sensitivity to peanut is generally lifelong.[42] Children who develop IgE-mediated food allergy after 3 years of age are less likely to lose their sensitivity than children who show symptoms in infancy.[43]

A skilled nutritionist will also teach the patient to recognize the offending product and its derivatives on food labels and to remain aware of the possible ingredient changes in the processed foods.[21,44] The Food Allergy Network provides public awareness and patient education support. Patients can obtain a personalized emergency care card from the Network and should be encouraged to wear a bracelet engraved with emergency phone numbers and the allergenic food. Such a bracelet can be obtained from the Medic Alert Foundation. Ultimately, the first line of defense against an allergic reaction is the education the patient has received. (Table 3–10). When the reaction is life-threatening, the patient must be taught how to use, and be equipped with, a readily available dose of injectable adrenaline or epinephrine and precalculated doses of drinkable antihistamine and steroids. Children can be encouraged to carry these medications at all times, when away from their

Table 3–10   Help Available to Patients with Food Allergies
The Food Allergy Network 4744 Holly Avenue Fairfax, VA 22030–5647 703–691–3179 Fax 703–691–2713 Medic Alert Foundation International: 800–344–3226 National Institutes of Health Medicine for the Public Food Allergy and Intolerances Publication No. 93–3469 April 1993

parents, in an inconspicuous or fashionable waist pouch. However, patients should still seek medical attention after using their emergency treatment.

When strict avoidance of the allergenic food cannot be adhered to, or the response to the elimination diet remains suboptimal, or the agent causing the IgE-mediated reaction has eluded all diagnostic means, it would be tempting to turn to daily medication. However, disodium cromoglycate, taken orally, has shown little effectiveness; chronically administered steroids have unacceptable side effects; and antihistamines, helpful in hiding some cutaneous symptoms, cannot control the full extent of respiratory and gastro-intestinal manifestations of immediate food allergy.[45] Oral ketotifen and prostaglandin synthetase inhibitors are being studied and show promise.

Immunotherapy has been attempted and although the reaction rate has been much higher than observed in aero-allergen desensitization, patients have shown significant reduction in their reactivity. This method is still investigational.[46] Oral and sublingual desensitization techniques at this time have no place in the armamentarium against IgE-mediated food allergy.[47]

Prevention

The question of preventing or only postponing the expression of atopic manifestations by the manipulation of the mother's diet during pregnancy and lactation and the child's alimentation during infancy and the first few years of life is still unanswered. Breast milk should be the preferred alimentation during the first 6 months of life, leaving this period, as much as possible, free of allergen exposure. Furthermore, if it is determined that the child is at high risk for atopy—having two parents or one parent and one sibling with atopy[48,49]—the mother should try to avoid highly allergenic foods (milk, egg, and peanut) in her diet while breastfeeding, because minute amounts of allergens present in her milk can sensitize the infant. These restrictions do not seem warranted during pregnancy at this time.

As a general recommendation, solid foods should not be introduced before 6 months of age, and children at high risk should not take cow's milk before 12 months, unless in the form of a hypoallergenic, highly hydrolyzed, cow's milk protein supplement; eggs until 2 or 3 years; and peanuts, nuts, and seafood until 3 or 4 years of age. These diet adjustments seem to delay the expression of the genetically determined atopic syndrome.[50,51] The length of this delay has yet to be determined.[52]

References

1. Metcalfe DD. Food hypersensitivity. *J Allergy Clin Immunol* 1984;73:749.
2. Bock SA. Prospective appraisal of complaints of adverse reactions to foods in children during the first three years of life. *Pediatrics* 1987;79:683–688.
3. Anderson JA, Sogn DD, eds. Adverse reactions to foods. AAAAI and NIAID, NIH Publication No. 84–2442, 1984.
4. Brunzeel-Koomen C, Ortolani C. Position paper of the European Academy of Allergy and Clinical Immunology on Adverse Reactions to Food, 1994.
5. Blaylock WK. Atopic dermatitis: diagnosis and pathobiology. *J Allergy Clin Immunol* 1976;57:62–79.
6. Burks AW, Mallory SB, Williams LW, Shirrell MA. Atopic dermatitis: clinical relevance of food hypersensitivity reactions. *J Pediatr* 1988;113:447–451.
7. Sampson HA. The role of food allergy and mediator release in atopic dermatitis. *J Allergy Clin Immunol* 1988;81:635–645.
8. Chan-Yeung M, Malo JL. Current concepts. Occupational asthma. *Current Concepts* 1994;333(2):107–112.
9. Onorato J, Merland N, Terral C, Michael FB, Bousquet J. Placebo-controlled double-blind food challenge in asthma. *J Allergy Clin Immunol* 1986;78:1139–1146.
10. Sampson HA, Metcalfe DD. Immediate reactions to foods. In: Metcalfe DD, Sampson HA, Simon RA, eds. *Food Allergy: Adverse Reactions to Foods and Food Additives*. Boston, Mass: Blackwell Scientific Publications, 1991;99–112.
11. Fink JN. Hypersensitivity pneumonitis. In: Lynch JP, DeRemee RA, eds. *Immunologically Mediated Pulmonary Diseases*. Philadelphia, Pa: JB Lippincott; 1991:399–412.
12. Champion RH, Robert SO, Carpenter RG, Roger JH. Urticaria and angioedema; a review of 554 patients. *Br J Dermatol* 1969;81:558–597.
13. Winton GB, Lewis CW. Contact urticaria. *Int J Dermatol* 1982;21:573–578.
14. Enberg RN. Food-induced oropharyngeal symptoms: the oral allergy syndrome. In: Anderson JA, ed. *Food Allergy: Immunology and Allergy Clinics of North America*. Philadelphia, Pa: WB Saunders Co, 1991;11:767–772.
15. Ortolani C, Ispano M, Pastorello EA, et al. The oral allergy syndrome. *Ann Allergy* 1988;61:47.
16. Bircher AJ, Van Mell G, Haller E, et al. IgE to food allergens are highly prevalent in patients allergic to pollens, with and without symptoms of food allergy. *Clin Exp Allergy* 1994;24:367.
17. Min K, Metcalfe DD. Eosinophilic gastroenteritis. *Immunol Allergy Clin North Am* 1991;11:799–814.
18. Sampson HA. Infantile colic and food allergy: fact or fiction. *J Pediatr* 1989;115:583–584.
19. Taylor SL, Busse WW, Sachs MI, Parker JL, Yunginger JW. Peanut oil is not allergenic to peanut-sensitive individuals. *J Allergy Clin Immunol* 1981;68:372–375.
20. Bush RK, Taylor SL, Nordlee JA, Busse WW. Soybean oil is not allergenic to soybean-sensitive individuals. *J Allergy Clin Immunol* 1985;76:242–245.
21. Porras O, Carlsson B, Fallstrom SP, Hanson LA. Detection of soy protein in soy lecithin, margarine and occasionally soy oil. *Int Arch Allergy Immunol* 1985;78:30–32.
22. Sampson HA. Food allergy and the role of immunotherapy. Editorial. *J Allergy Clin Immunol* 1992;151–152.

23. Bernhisel-Broadbent J. Allergenic cross-reactivity of foods and characterization of food allergens and extracts. *Ann Allergy Asthma Immunol* 1995;75:295–304.
24. Bock SA, Atkins FM. Patterns of food hypersensitivity during sixteen years of double-blind placebo-controlled food challenges. *J Pediatr* 1990;117:561–567.
25. Bernhisel-Broadbent J, Sampson HA. Cross-allergenicity in the legume botanical family in children with food hypersensitivity. *J Allergy Clin Immunol* 1989;83:435–40.
26. Bernhisel-Broadbent J, Taylor S, Sampson HA. Cross-allergenicity in the legume botanical family in children with food hypersensitivity. II. Laboratory correlates. *J Allergy Clin Immunol* 1989;84:701–709.
27. Jones SM, Cooke K, Sampson HA. Immunologic cross-reactivity among cereal grains and grasses in children with food hypersensitivity. *J Allergy Clin Immunol* 1993;81:343. Abstract.
28. Daul CB, Morgan JE, Lehrer SB. The natural history of shrimp hypersensitivity. *J Allergy Clin Immunol* 1990;86:88–93.
29. Bernhisel-Broadbent J, Sampson HA. Fish hypersensitivity. I. Laboratory studies and oral challenges in fish allergic patients. *J Allergy Clin Immunol* 1991;89:730–737.
30. Haydel R, El-Dahr J, McCants M, et al. Food allergy: challenge studies of fish allergic subjects. *J Allergy Clin Immunol* 1993;91:344. Abstract.
31. Van Ree R, Aalberse R. Pollen-vegetable cross-reactivity: serological and clinical relevance of cross-reacting IgE. *J Clin Immunoassay* 1993;16:124.
32. Pastorello EA, Ortolani C, Farioli L, et al. Allergenic cross-reactivity among peach, apricot, plum, and cherry in patients with oral allergy syndrome. An in vivo and in vitro study. *J Allergy Clin Immunol* 1994;94:699–707.
33. Bernstein IL, Storms WW. Practice parameters for allergy diagnostic testing. *Ann Allergy Asthma Immunol* 1995;75:6–587.
34. Pastorello EA, Stocchi L, Pravetonni V, et al. Role of the elimination diet in adults with food allergy. *J Allergy Clin Immunol* 1989;84:475–483.
35. Bock SA, Sampson HA, Atkins FM, et al. Double-blind placebo-controlled food challenge (DBPCFC) as an office procedure; a manual. *J Allergy Clin Immunol* 1988;82:986.
36. Dohi M, Suko M, Sugiyami H, et al. Food-dependent, exercise-induced anaphylaxis: a study of 11 Japanese cases. *J Allergy Clin Immunol* 1991;87:34–40.
37. Sampson HA. Comparative study of commercial food antigen extracts for the diagnosis of food hypersensitivity. *J Allergy Clin Immunol* 1988;82:718–726.
38. Treveno AJ, Rapaport S. Problems with in vitro diagnosis of food allergy. *ENT Journal* 1990;1:69.
39. Reimann HJ, Ring J, Ultsch B, Wendt P. Intragastric provocation under endoscopic control (IPEC) in food allergy: mast cell and histamine change in gastric mucosa. *Clin Allergy* 1985;15:195–202.
40. Moon A, Kleinman RE. Allergic gastroenteropathy in children. *Ann Allergy Asthma Immunol* 1995;74:5–12.
41. Barnes-Koerner C, Sampson HA. Diets and nutrition food allergy. In: Metcalfe DD, Sampson HA, Simon RA, eds. *Food Allergy: Adverse Reactions to Foods and Food Additives.* Boston: Blackwell Scientific Publications; 1991;332–354.
42. Bock SA, Atkins FM. The natural history of peanut allergy. *J Allergy Clin Immunol* 1989;83:900–904.
43. Bock SA. The natural history of food hypersensitivity. *J Allergy Clin Immunol* 1982;69:173–177.
44. Gern J, Sampson HA. Allergic reactions to milk-contaminated "non-dairy" products. *N Engl J Med* 1991;324:976–979.
45. Sogn DD. Medications and their use in the treatment of adverse reactions to foods. *J Allergy Clin Immunol* 1986;78:238–243.
46. Oppenheimer JJ, Nelson HS, Bock SA, et al. Treatment of peanut allergy with rush immunotherapy. *J Allergy Clin Immunol* 1992;90:256–262.
47. Sampson HA, Metcalfe DD. Food allergies. In: *Primer on Allergic and Immunologic Diseases,* Chapter 6, deShazo RD and Smith DL, eds. *JAMA* 1992;268(20):2840–2844.
48. Zeiger RS, Heller S, Mellon MH, et al. Effect of combined maternal and infant food-allergen avoidance on development of atopy in early infancy: a randomized study. *J Allergy Clin Immunol* 1989;84:72–89.
49. Kellman NIM. Epidemiology of food allergy. In: Schmidt E, Reinhardt MC, eds. *Food Allergy.* New York: Raven Press; 1988;301.
50. Zeiger RS, Heller S, Mellon MH, et al. Effect of combined maternal and infant food-allergen

avoidance on development of atopy in early infancy: a randomized study. *J Allergy Clin Immunol* 1989;84:72–89.
51. Zeiger RS, Heller S, Mellon MH, Halsey JF, Hamburger RN, Sampson HA. Genetic and environmental factors affecting the development of atopy through age 4 in children of atopic parents: a prospective randomized study of food allergen avoidance. *Pediatr Allergy Immunol* 1992;3:110–127.
52. Hide DW, Matthews S, Matthews L, Stevens M, Ridout S, Twiselton R, Gant C, Arshad SH. Effect of allergen avoidance in infancy on allergic manifestations at age two years. *J Allergy Clin Immunol* 1994;93:842–846.

◆ 4 ◆

Food Allergy—Signs and Symptoms

Hamilton S. Dixon, M.D.

The signs and symptoms of food allergy are frequently overlooked by both patient and physician. Such signs and symptoms may have multiple possible causes. The least likely of these causes often require expensive workups. In many cases, the most common cause is food allergy. The proper identification of the offending food can be very effective from the standpoint of cost and of returning the patient to full productivity.

The difference between immediate and delayed allergy is especially important in diagnosing food sensitivities. Whereas IgE mediates immediate reactions, including anaphylaxis, type III mechanisms are largely responsible for delayed reactions, mediated mainly by IgG, representing an immune complex disease.[1] Type II antibody-dependent cytotoxicity has been reported in vitro with sera from infants with cow's milk protein–induced gastroenteropathy.[2] Type IV cell-mediated responses have been shown to be at least indirectly involved in delayed allergy to gliadin, a prolamine contained in gluten, involved in celiac disease.[3,4] Immediate-type food allergies are often known to the patient and family, but delayed food allergy has no apparent cause-and-effect relationship, because of the elapsed time as well as the mix of foods ingested. Because delayed allergy is both time- and dose-dependent,[1] symptoms are intermittent and often masked.[5] When people have had certain subtle and intermittent symptoms for many years, blame is sidetracked to stress, working too hard, the side effects of medication, and other unrelated causes. When symptoms become severe and interfere with normal activities, physicians must have the tools available to diagnose the correct cause.

IgE allergy is almost always repeatable, but the signs and symptoms of delayed food allergy do not follow the usual repeatability accepted as a scientific principle of biologic systems. For example, a given food might be eaten on several consecutive days and produce no recognized symptoms. The patient might then unknowingly omit that particular food for 4 or 5 days, and be set up for a faster and more recognizable reaction because of being at the peak of food intolerance on that day, the hyperreactive phase of cyclic food allergy.[6] This time, the same ingested food, at the same dose, causes significant and recognizable symptoms according to which shock organs are involved. Because the food was known to be eaten on prior days and caused no symptoms, the allergy remains undiagnosed by the physician or patient. This is explained by the concept of cyclic food allergy. As the food antigens are cleared with elimination after 4–5 days, high levels of IgG antibodies are still being produced; the food immune complexes become insoluble and are deposited on sensitized cells. If a large amount of the food antigen is then introduced on the fifth day during this hyperacute phase, significant symptoms can occur with considerable mediator release. These insoluble complexes are also associated with withdrawal symptoms that also lead the patient to reintroduce a much larger quantity of the food (without realizing what is really happening).[7]

If the food is withheld beyond this hyperacute phase, the food immune complexes are gradually metabolized as tolerance to the food antigen begins. Within 5 to 6 months, the IgG antibodies are finally gone and tolerance is complete.[1]

Food sensitivity can affect virtually any organ system in the body.[8] Signs and symptoms depend entirely on which shock organ is sensitized; multiple organ systems are often involved. Because food is ingested into the gastrointestinal tract, GI symptoms should be the first consideration in deciding whether food allergy could be a significant problem. If most of the typical gastrointestinal symptoms are insignificant, the likelihood of delayed food allergy is not great. However, this may not be true for immediate food allergies, particularly for patients who have multiple severe sensitivities, such as asthma and hives.[9]

The following list of conditions is offered as a guide in considering the possibility of food allergy.

1. Only 50% improvement on immunotherapy after 2 months*
2. Negative RAST or skin tests in patients with multiple allergy symptoms
3. "Functional GI symptoms," gas, belching, fatigue after meals, intermittent diarrhea, bloating, cramps, indigestion, and alternating diarrhea and constipation
4. GERDS (gastroesophageal reflux distress syndrome)
5. Peptic ulcers

* Based on modified radioallergosorbent test (RAST) or skin endpoint titration[10] and initiating therapy at the end-point dilution.

6. Irritable bowel syndrome
7. Crohn's disease
8. Celiac disease
9. Ulcerative colitis
10. Spastic colon
11. Recurrent diarrhea (with other causes ruled out)
12. Atopic dermatitis
13. Chronic itching
14. Urticaria
15. Angioedema
16. Eczema
17. Psoriasis
18. Dermatitis herpetiformis
19. Allergic conjunctivitis
20. Eyelid itching
21. Benign paroxysmal positional vertigo
22. Meniere's disorder
23. Tinnitus (with normal hearing; other causes ruled out)
24. Fluctuating sensorineural hearing loss (cochlear hydrops)
25. Chronic secretory otitis media
26. Recurrent suppurative otitis media
27. Chronic otitis media and mastoiditis with or without cholesteatoma
28. Eczematoid otitis externa
29. Recurrent fungal otitis externa
30. Allergic rhinitis (with "functional GI symptoms") or with negative tests for inhalant allergy
31. Turbinate hypertrophy with nasal airway obstruction
32. Nasal polyps
33. Upper airway resistance syndrome with turbinate hypertrophy
34. Obstructive sleep apnea with swollen turbinates, long swollen uvula, low swollen palate, high tongue, etc.
35. Recurrent sinusitis
36. Chronic sinusitis
37. Sinus polyps
38. Aphthous ulcers
39. Oral allergy syndrome
40. Recurrent sore throats without fever
41. Clicking of the palate (clonic contractions of the uvula)
42. Frequent throat clearing
43. "Lump in the throat" sensation (globus syndrome)
44. Intermittent hoarseness with "normal vocal folds" at indirect laryngoscopy ("functional dysphonia")
45. Polypoid swelling of vocal folds
46. Vocal fold nodule that is actually small, soft polypoid swelling
47. Rienke's edema of vocal folds (with nicotine abuse)

48. Cough (nonproductive)
49. Asthma
50. Asthmatic bronchitis
51. Mental dullness (unexplained)
52. Mood swings
53. Forgetfulness
54. Depression aggravated and worsened by food allergy
55. Decreased libido (associated with other signs and symptoms of food allergy)
56. Muscle spasm
57. Myalgia
58. Cervical muscle contraction headaches
59. Sinus headaches
60. Migraine headaches
61. Horton's histamine cephalgia
62. Chronic fatigue
63. Chronic monilial allergy ("chronic candidiasis") and chronic fatigue syndrome
64. Edema
65. Weight fluctuation and intermittent swelling (idiopathic cyclic edema)
66. Idiopathic "anaphylaxis," "pseudoanaphylaxis"
67. Tachycardia (unexplained and with other signs and symptoms of food allergy)
68. Cardiac rhythm disturbances (when other signs and symptoms of food allergy are present and when cardiac workup negative for intrinsic disease)

A questionnaire has been expanded by the author to aid in identifying those patients who might have delayed food allergy as a significant problem (Table 4–1). The standard Candida Questionnaire and Score Sheet[11] for chronic monilial allergy is given to all patients who suffer from moderate to severe chronic fatigue, a symptom often overlooked on initial history taking. The built-in scoring system aids in deciding whether to pursue that possibility as well.

Gastrointestinal Symptoms

Gastrointestinal symptoms of delayed food allergy are referred to as *functional GI symptoms* by the gastroenterologist. In order of frequency, they are gas, belching, fatigue after meals, intermittent diarrhea, bloating, cramps, indigestion, and alternating diarrhea and constipation. These are all common gastrointestinal symptoms of delayed food allergy.[12] The presence of several of these symptoms can steer one to further investigate this possibility.

Infant colic is an indication of intestinal gas and abdominal cramps. This

---
Table 4–1   Food Allergy Questionnaire
INSTRUCTIONS
---

1. Answer all questions—be sure to enter the date and your name.

2. Be sure to circle numbers or letters in the left-hand margin for every question as follows:
   1 = Frequently
   2 = Occasionally
   3 = Never
   4 = Yes
   5 = No

3. Be certain to fill in all blanks unless the answer is No or Never.

4. These questions should be answered as an average over the past several months, not just the past 2 weeks.

5. Even if you think you know the cause of these symptoms in your case, still answer "YES" and explain.

6. Even if you have any of these symptoms and think they are normal, still answer "YES" and explain.

7. Please review these instructions again after you are finished to be sure all the blanks are filled in correctly.

CIRCLE ANSWER   BEGIN QUESTIONNAIRE

Y   N   1. What foods do you crave *or* eat often? (Example: More than one glass of Coke, tea, or milk a day.)
_____
_____

Y   N   2. Do any foods make you sick or disagree with you? Please list them.
_____
_____

1   2   3   3. Are you EVER awakened between the hours of 1:00 A.M. and 5:00 A.M. with the following symptoms: Headache, dizziness, stomach cramps, bloating, heartburn, or dry cough? (Circle 1, 2, or 3 and WRITE IN YOUR SYMPTOMS.)
_____

Y   N   4. Does any member of your family have hay fever, asthma, hives, chronic skin condition, migraine headache, dizziness, stomach cramps, bloating, dry cough or sinus condition? Answer Yes or No, then circle the condition(s). Which family member(s)?
_____

Table 4–1 Continued

Y N 5. During childhood, did you have any of the following: Eczema, hay fever, sinus trouble, asthma, or frequent earaches? (Circle which condition.)

Y N 6. Were you told that you had colic feeding problems as a baby?

1 2 3 7. Do you have itching of the skin, palate, or roof of mouth? (Circle 1, 2, or 3 and write in area of body affected.)

_____

_____

How often does it occur? _____

1 2 3 8. Do you notice swelling of the ankles, feet, hands, or face on arising in the morning? (Circle 1, 2, or 3 and write in area of body.)

_____

_____

1 2 3 9. After a full meal in the middle of the day, do you *ever* experience sleepiness or fatigue 1–2 hours later? Even if you usually eat only a snack for lunch, please choose a time when you would eat a full meal in the middle of the day (Example: After church on Sunday).

1 2 3 10. Do you experience a dry cough? How many coughs in 24 hours?

_____

_____

1 2 3 11. Do you eat snacks frequently between meals? What? (Circle 1, 2, or 3 and answer question.)

_____

_____

1 2 3 12. Do you have excessive chilling when a sudden change in temperature occurs?

1 2 3 13. Do you have migraine headaches? How often?

_____

_____

1 2 3 14. Do you have sinus headaches? How often?

_____

1 2 3 15. Do you have headaches in the back of your head? How often?

_____

1 2 3 16. Do you *ever* experience gas, bloating, abdominal distention, or cramps? (Circle the symptoms.) How often? _____

_____

1 2 3 17. Have you noticed numbness of the face, arms, or legs at periodic intervals with no apparent cause? (Circle which area.) How often? _____

_____

Table 4–1   Continued

1	2	3	18.	Do you have drowsiness, headache, or bloating following the ingestion of a cocktail or glass of beer or wine?
Y	N		19.	Are you allergic to penicillin?
1	2	3	20.	Do you *ever* have any diarrhea, even mild or intermittently? How often?
Y	N		21.	Do you *ever* experience repeated symptoms on awaking in the morning such as headache? Can you make the headache go away by eating or drinking any particular food such as coffee or Coke? What food helps to improve the symptoms?
Y	N		22.	Are there any other reactions or problems you notice with any other particular food? If, so, please list.
1	2	3	23.	Do you *ever* clear your throat? How many times per day?
Y	N		24.	Have you *ever* had dizziness? Episodic? Spinning by spells? Positional? When you move? How long does the average episode last?
Y	N		25.	Does your weight fluctuate? How many pounds in one week?

has been presumed to be an IgE-mediated phenomenon.[13] However, in the light of the material presented here, the likelihood of IgG delayed food sensitivity is high. These babies are more likely to develop recurrent otitis media and/or recurrent sinusitis. It is the proposition here that cyclic or delayed food allergy may be the major cause, and esophagal reflux may be an important additional factor.

Fatigue after meals is a common food allergy symptom, but is usually denied or not recognized by the patient. The approach to questioning a patient is the key to the correct answer. The average person with postprandial fatigue answers "no" when asked if he experiences fatigue after meals. If, however, one focuses on a specific time at which a normal full meal is eaten, especially midday, more accurate answers can be obtained.

Example

Mrs. Jones answered "NO" to this question on the questionnaire.

"Mrs. Jones, do you ever eat a full, regular meal in the middle of the day—for example, on the weekends or after church on Sunday?"
"Yes."

"Do you ever get sleepy or tired within an hour or two after eating this regular midday meal?"
"Yes."
"Are those symptoms frequent, occasional, or rare after a full meal?"
"Frequent."
"Do you avoid eating very much at lunch because you know it will make you sleepy?"
"Yes."

Therefore, getting an accurate and informed answer depends entirely on whether or not the patient fully understands the question and concentrates on the time period in which symptoms occur (Table 4–2). Busy people who live with these recurrent problems do not admit to these symptoms because to them the symptoms are normal. People who experience gas will frequently say *no* when asked. To them it is normal to have gas, and they think that you mean "more than normal." One must re-ask the question, "Do you *ever* have any gas on your stomach?" The difference is very revealing. Unfortunately, it takes the physician's personal time to obtain the correct answers to these questions, even after the nurse has done the initial history. If the questionnaire is mostly negative, re-asking questions 9, 16, and 20 may be helpful.

Skin

The skin is one of the most frequent target organs in food allergy. Itching and burning of the skin are more frequently associated with food allergy than with inhalant allergy.[14]

Ingested food antigens represent macromolecules and can cross the gastrointestinal barrier intact in the food-allergic patient, rapidly reaching inflammatory cells in the skin.[15] This may provoke urticaria and angioedema, atopic dermatitis, eczema, dermatitis herpetiformis or psoriasis. The transport of

Table 4–2   Food-Related Allergic Responses—Gastrointestinal

SYMPTOMS	SIGNS
Gas (flatus)	Infant colic
Fatigue after meals	Eructation
Belching	Postprandial abdominal swelling
Cramps	Loose stools
Intermittent diarrhea	Increased bowel sounds
Alternating diarrhea and constipation	Diarrhea
Heartburn	Increased gastric acid
Indigestion	Inflammation of gastric or
Epigastric pain	esophagal mucosa

these macromolecules leads to a relatively rapid onset of symptoms (Table 4–3).

Eczema

Atopic dermatitis is a form of eczema characterized by extreme pruritus and typical distribution; it may be associated with asthma and allergic rhinitis.[16]
Eczema is an extension of mold as well as food allergy and affects the skin with itching and dry, scaly eruptions. Eczematoid external otitis is a characteristic dry, scaly condition of the ear canals that can flare up with swelling, weeping, exudate, and fungal infection. When this is recurrent, TOE (trichophyton, oidiomyces, epidermophyton) can be tested, but foods may also be part of the problem.[17]

Urticaria and Angioedema

When food allergen–specific IgE is bound to cutaneous mast cells, food antigens are absorbed and rapidly transported to the skin. Various foods, such as shellfish, have been incriminated in these conditions,[18,19] but it has been the author's experience that hidden foods such as milk, wheat, corn, egg, and peanut may be more often responsible for the urticaria and angioedema. This is often cyclic food allergy of short delay. Chronic urticaria was not found to be caused by IgE-mediated food allergy,[20] but delayed allergy was also studied. In recurrent acute urticaria and angioedema especially, a type III delayed reaction with complement cascade may be a more important mechanism than the presumed IgE. This is evidenced by a history of many recurrent episodes that do not get worse, and a poor response to epinephrine injections.[21] Immediate as well as delayed food hypersensitivity, plus the likelihood of mold allergy, can be a causative factor. Urticaria is a sign of intradermal histamine release and can be caused by many incitants. Urticaria and angioedema respond well to intravenous heparin, which binds serotonin and prevents the release of histamine.[22]

Table 4–3   Food-Related Allergic Responses—Skin

SYMPTOMS	SIGNS
Itching	Rash
Breaking out	Urticaria
Swelling	Erythema
Whelps	Angioedema
Welts	Dry scaling
Hives	Fissuring and weeping
Dryness	Crusts
Cracking	
Scabs (drying of serous exudate)	
Burning	
Pain	

Eyes

Dark circles under the eyes may represent congenital pigmentation as well as allergy, chronic sinus infection, and chronic fatigue. Only when all diagnoses are exhausted does one look to find other reasons, such as food allergy. Though watering and redness of the eyes are usually associated with pollen, dust, and mold allergy, some patients have these symptoms when certain foods are ingested.

The "red eye" of allergic origin is classified by clinical criteria. Allergic conjunctivitis, the most common, can be seasonal or perennial and is not serious. Vernal keratoconjunctivitis is much worse, and is IgE-mediated in only one half the cases. Corneal involvement can develop if the condition is not controlled. Atopic keratoconjunctivitis is associated with eczema of the eyelids, and complications are more frequent (Table 4–4). Atopic eczema is often related to food allergy, as is atopic keratoconjunctivitis. Non–IgE-mediated triggering of mast cells and basophils can be induced by anaphylatoxins C3a and C5a, ILs, and so on, and has been referred to as pseudo-allergic reactions. These are clinically very similar to classical IgE reactions,[23] and delayed food allergy can be a part of this process.

Table 4–4   Food-related Allergic Response—Eye

SYMPTOMS	SIGNS
Allergic Conjunctivitis	
Tearing	Mild hyperemia
Burning	Mild eczema
Mild itching	Mild papillary reaction
Blurred vision	
Vernal Keratoconjunctivitis	
Intense itching	Cobblestone papillae
Tearing	Intense hyperemia
Photophobia	Mucus discharge
Sensation of foreign body	Milky conjunctivae
Blurred vision	Punctate keratopathy
	Tranta's dots
	Togley's ulcers
Atopic Keratoconjunctivitis	
Itching	Hyperemia
Burning	Eczematoid lesions of eyelids
Tearing	Corneal ulcers
Blurred vision	Cataracts
Blindness	Pannus
	Keratoconus
	Retinal detachment

Ears

Itchy ear canals are often associated with mold as well as food allergy. When the mold-type foods such as cheese and mushrooms are ingested, the itching ear symptoms can increase (see eczema).

Though one normally does not think of hearing loss as a food allergy symptom, there are several situations in which hearing loss is found in conjunction with food allergy. Food sensitivity can cause eustachian tube edema and obstruction, with resulting negative pressure, middle ear fluid, and subsequent conductive hearing loss.

Recurrent otitis media in childhood is a common problem. Risk factors have been studied,[24] but pediatricians and pediatric-allergists alike have been discouraged about testing these children for allergy. It has been said that allergy is rarely the cause of recurrent otitis media or otitis media with effusion.[25] These studies have been based on traditional skin tests for dust, molds, and foods, but have not included tests for delayed food allergy. The incidence of repeat ventilation tubes drops dramatically when RAST for dust and molds is combined with tests for delayed food allergy with subsequent specific treatment of inhalants and total elimination of positive foods.[26–28]

Though there are no conclusive studies showing that sensorineural hearing loss is caused by food allergy, the elimination of allergenic foods has definitely been shown to relieve tinnitus in some patients.[29] Elimination of an offending food has stopped attacks of vertigo in certain patients with Meniere's syndrome, with subsequent improvement in hearing.[30,31] Delayed food allergy is now implicated in as many as two thirds of patients with Meniere's syndrome. An increase in circulating immune complexes has been shown in patients with Meniere's syndrome and has been linked to immune-complex disease.[32] In cochlear hydrops, if an offending food can be correctly identified, the fluctuating sensorineural hearing loss may be improved or stopped. Elimination of an offending food can even avoid the need for endolymphatic shunt surgery in those so afflicted.[21]

There are three possible roles for allergy in the production of fluid in the endolymphatic sac (ES) leading to Meniere's disease.[33]

1. The ES may be a target organ of mediator release from inhalant or food reactions. The blood supply to the sac is unique, coming from the posterior meningeal artery of the occipital branch of the external carotid artery. These arteriolar branches are fenestrated and "leaky," making them vulnerable to vasoactive mediators such as histamine.
2. Circulating immune complexes to a food or inhalant antigen are deposited in the sac through these fenestrated vessels, causing inflammation. This interferes with the sac's filtering capability, resulting in toxic accumulation of metabolic products that interferes with hair cell function. These antigen–antibody complexes localized in and around the perisaccular vascular walls induce an inflammatory response mediated through complement

activation and by the influx of phagocytic cells. Chemotactic factors promote the migration of polymorphs and macrophages into this area. These complexes bind to cell membranes, facilitating phagocytosis with the release of tissue-damaging enzymes.

3. There is a proposed viral antigen/allergic interaction.[24] IgG, M, and A antibody titers to viral infection in childhood—including rubeola, varicella, mumps, HSV-1, CMV, and rubella—have all been shown to be elevated in patients with Meniere's syndrome compared with control subjects.[35] This can cause a mild impairment in sac absorption. Later, if an excess in endolymphatic fluid is produced by an allergic reaction, the "sick sac" cannot compensate, and endolymphatic hydrops results.

When patients present with typical benign paroxysmal positional vertigo—and have the "extralabyrinthine symptoms" of delayed food allergy (functional GI symptoms including gas, belching, bloating, occasional diarrhea, fatigue after meals, etc)—delayed food allergy may be related to the cause.[21] The simple procedure of placing the patient on a "caveman diet" (Table 4–5) for 2 weeks may clear the vertigo and negate the need for an expensive neuro-otologic workup including audiologic evaluation, ABR, ENG, and CT or MRI scans. If the patient is 50% improved or better in 2 weeks, proceeding with specific food allergy diagnosis is reasonable. Naturally, careful follow-up is required. An appropriate neuro-otologic workup may be ordered at any time when indicated (Table 4–6).

Table 4–5   Caveman Diet

I. Eat all you want of:
Fresh fruits (frozen, if home prepared, or in plastic bags from grocery store).
Fresh vegetables (or as above).
Broiled, boiled, or baked meat, but do not eat any meat more than one time per day.
Drink pure fruit juice, vegetable juice, and water (bottled or filtered is better)

II. You may not have any prepared food products (boxed mixes, etc)
You may not have cake, cookies, candy, or soft drinks.
You may not have any grains or nuts (including rice and soy).
You may not have any dairy products—milk, butter, margarine, cheese, yogurt, ice cream, etc.
You may not have any fruit, vegetable, or meat to which you have been found allergic.
Fruit "drinks" contain corn syrup and are *NOT* allowed.

III. You may have one teaspoon of honey per day.

IV. Corn—even though often considered a vegetable—is a grain, and is to be totally eliminated.

V. The purpose of this diet is to get the "hidden foods" out of the diet: corn, eggs, wheat, milk, sugar, soy, peanut, as well as chocolate, coffee, etc. These are the foods that people are most likely allergic to.

Table 4–6   **Food-Related Allergic Responses—EAR**

SYMPTOMS	SIGNS
Clear or purulent drainage	Dry canal skin without cerumen formation
Itching	Scaly red skin
Irritation	Swollen canal skin
Fullness	Swollen canal skin with cheesy-white exudate
Pressure	Redness and fissuring in postauricular fold
Popping	Clear otorrhea
Ringing	Hearing loss:
Off balance	conductive
Hearing loss	• fluid in middle ears with many different
Pain	possibilities of tympanic membrane
Clicking	presentations—
Positional vertigo	• retracted
Episodic vertigo	• fluid bubbles with double refractile lines
Dizziness	• amber color
Floating	• slate blue with a chalky white malleus
	handle
	• prominent short process of malleus due
	to retraction
	• radial injection of annulus
	• opaque
	• normal
	sensorineural
	• low tone
	• fluctuating
	Findings on electronystagmography:
	• peripheral-type positional nystagmus
	• spontaneous nystagmus
	• directional preponderance
	Impedence audiometry findings of spontaneous
	stapedial reflex jerks associated with
	"clicking" reports by patient

Nose

Nasal obstruction can be related to food allergy causing swelling of the turbinates. Pollen, dust, and mold allergies are the cause of allergic rhinitis in 80% of allergic adults, but in 20% of those patients food allergy plays a significant role. In 5% of patients, food allergy may be the major factor.[21] Controlled food challenges in infants with rhinitis showed cow's milk allergy in 21%[36] and 39%.[37] In older children, allergy to various foods, including milk, is reported in up to 39%.[38] The prevalence of rhinitis confirmed by double-blind placebo-controlled food challenges in adults is reported to be from 0% to 80%.[39]

Children may have a ridge just above the tip of the nose caused by the "allergic salute." This is due to intense itching of the nostrils and columella. Stretching the nasal tip upward pulls on the attachments to the nasal spine, similar to pressing on the spine. This gives some temporary relief (firm pressure on the nasal spine also stops an impending sneeze). The mucus membrane lining of the nose and sinuses produces a quart of mucus every 24 hours. The cilia beat toward the nasopharynx, moving the mucus blanket posteriorly, which is then swallowed. This self-cleansing mechanism is disturbed by allergy, and mucus can increase up to 2 to 3 quarts per day. There is a sol layer under and a gel layer on the surface that the cilia engage to move the mucus.[40] When mucus becomes too thick, the cilia are not strong enough to move it along, and the material stagnates, becomes secondarily infected, and turns yellow. Thick mucus causes an annoying postnasal drip that does not drain normally. The cause of this increase in the gel layer has not been explained, but it has been shown clinically in some patients that delayed food allergy is related.[21] This problem has a profound effect on the cause of chronic sinusitis. Frequent swallowing and clearing the throat are ineffective in clearing thick postnasal drip. Much worse is the thick, stagnated secretions at the sinus ostia.

Sniffing, sneezing, snorting, and blowing the nose may represent immediate as well as delayed food reactions (Table 4–7).

Almost any symptom one sees with dust, mold, or pollen allergy can also be present in the patient who is allergic to a particular food. As a matter of fact, because of concomitant food allergy and the total allergic load principle,[11] these symptoms to foods can occur during pollen season. For example, a patient with a concomitant allergy to wheat and pollen can tolerate wheat all year but becomes symptomatic in pollen season.[42,43]

Upper Airway Resistance Syndrome

Turbinate swelling due to allergy (including foods) causes nasal airway obstruction. This is more manifest in the supine position during sleep, which

Table 4–7 Food-Related Allergic Responses—NOSE

SYMPTOMS	SIGNS
Sniffing	Mouth breathing
Sneezing	Nasal obstruction
Snorting	Swelling of the turbinates
Blowing	Swelling of septal turbinates
Itching	Rhinorrhea
Mucus drainage (runny nose)	Sniffing
Blockage or obstruction to breathing (congestion)	Sneezing
Keeping a cold	Snorting
A cold that lingers	Blowing
	Ridge above tip secondary to "nasal salute" with redness of the columella and alae
	Nasal polyps
	"Adenoid facies" 2° to long-term nasal airway obstruction

insidiously causes a gradual increase in a set of symptoms. These go unrecognized by both the patient and physician. This is now referred to as *upper airway resistance syndrome.*[44] It begins as waking with a dry throat, progresses to waking fatigued, snoring, waking during sleep, and finally waking at night for water (Table 4–8). This, in the presence of additional circumstances such as a deviated nasal septum, low palate with a long uvula, high tongue, lack of exercise, and weight gain may lead to obstructive sleep apnea.

Obstructive Sleep Apnea

Nasal obstruction with turbinal hypertrophy is intermittent and may worsen insidiously. When people are young and healthy, they compensate well and often do not complain of nasal airway obstruction symptoms, such as waking with a dry throat. A deviated nasal septum adds significantly to this obstruction, and it is worse at night during sleep in the supine position. As aging continues, the ability to compensate diminishes. As activity diminishes and percent body fat increases, these same symptoms begin to constitute a sleep disorder. In those who have edema from delayed food allergy, particularly palate and uvular edema, snoring becomes worse and obstructive sleep apnea may develop. A protuberant abdomen is an additional significant

Table 4–8   Upper Airway Resistance Syndrome

SYMPTOMS	SIGNS
Waking in A.M. with dry throat	Rhinorrhea
Waking in A.M. tired	Restless sleep
Waking at night	turning frequently
Waking at night for water	leg kicking
Snoring	Snoring
Runny nose	Waking at night "in a jerk"
Blockage to breathing	Gasping for air
	Mouth breathing during sleep
	Deviated nasal septum
	Turbinate hypertrophy
	Adenoid hypertrophy or nasopharyngeal mass
	Intranasal mass
	polyps
	tumors
	Choanal atresia
	Purulent sinus drainage
	Adenoid facies
	Fragmented sleep—short alpha EEG arousals directly related to abnormal increase in respiratory effort on sleep study
	low palate
	long urula
	high tongue

factor. The weight of the abdominal contents in the supine position can only extend upward, compressing the diaphragm and thoracic cavity with increased venous pressure extending into the pharyngeal area. The tongue becomes larger and higher as the palate swells more and becomes relatively lower, with the swollen uvula filling the narrowed hypopharynx. Edema from allergy adds to this pathophysiology. This can make the difference between upper airway resistance syndrome with snoring and full-blown obstructive sleep apnea. Hypertension is a serious added factor that increases the risk of heart attack and stroke, and can lead to sudden death from sleep apnea.[45]

Sudden infant death syndrome has also been linked to pharyngeal airway obstruction. One author reported anaphylaxis to milk as the cause[46] (Table 4–9).

Sinuses

Sinus symptoms are caused by swelling of mucosa, increased or thickened mucus production, and obstruction.[47] Particularly in food allergy, the viscosity of mucus production can be increased, with decreased ciliary clearance. Pooling and stagnation of thick secretions lead to infection, which sets up a vicious circle of more swelling, obstruction, pain in the acute phase, and continued infection.[48]

The mechanism of sinus headaches is controversial. Pressure points with coaptation of mucosal surfaces with referred areas of pain in the head have

Table 4–9   Obstructive Sleep Apnea

SYMPTOMS	SIGNS
Waking fatigued	Noisy breathing
Daytime fatigue	Loud snoring
Daytime somnolence	Very restless sleep with accentuated leg and
falling asleep driving	body movements
Waking at night gasping for air	Apneic episodes during sleep of greater than
Waking with nightmares	10 seconds
	Hypopneas
	Decreased oxygen saturation
	Mouth breathing during sleep
	Low palate
	Hypertrophied uvula
	High tongue
	Weight gain
	Obesity
	Respiratory distress index on sleep study of
	10 or greater

Also see Tables 4–7, 4–8, and 4–10.

been reported.[49] Swelling from allergy can be a major factor. Acute obstruction of a sinus may cause pain as the result of rapid change in air pressure. Patients who can predict weather change have an osteomeatal complex that is congenitally narrow, and swelling from allergy, especially after food ingestion, causes even more obstruction. Barometric pressure change can then acutely obstruct the sinus, preventing equalization of air pressure as the barometer drops. Chronic obstruction often causes little or no pain, making chronic sinusitis impossible to diagnose without x-rays. If patients who have chronic sinusitis also have sinus headaches, some of them will be relieved by appropriate surgery and some will not.[21] Allergy is often an important factor in these patients, but inhalant allergy treatment alone may not help the headaches. Delayed food allergy, however, is often found to be the key factor in these sinus headaches. Complete relief often follows elimination of the allergic food (Table 4–10).

Mouth and Throat

The Oral Allergy Syndrome consists of tingling, pruritus, and angioedema of the lips, buccal mucosa, and pharynx after food ingestion. This is said to be IgE-mediated, with cross-reactivity with pollen allergens. Although IgG responses have been found, the exact mechanisms remain to be elucidated.[50]

Table 4–10   Food-Related Allergic Reponses—Sinus

SYMPTOMS	SIGNS
None admitted by patient	None
Nasal drainage	Turbinate hypertrophy
continous	Rhinorrhea
intermittent	clear anteriorly
Nasal obstruction	purulent drainage may be seen only
Fullness	with endoscope
Pain	Recurrent infections with purulent
Pressure	drainage
Sinus headaches	Chronic infection with continuous
Predicting weather change (feeling	purulent drainage
barometric pressure change)	Thick and/or purulent postnasal
Recurrent colds	drainage
Recurrent episodes of yellow drainage	Nasal polyps
Chronic yellow drainage	Mucosal thickening of low radiographic
"Keeping a cold"	density (edema of sinus mucosa)
A cold that lingers	Mucosal thickening of high radiographic
	density (infection)
	Sinus cyst seen radiographically
	Sinus polyps seen radiographically
	Fluid level of low radiographic density
	(mucoid fluid level)
	Fluid level of high density (pus)

Perioral rashes, fissuring of the mouth, and aphthous ulcers in the mouth and throat are all likely food-related allergic responses. A curious relationship between food sensitivity and the herpes virus has been observed for many years and is being studied.[34]

Many patients present to the physician with a "lump in the throat" (globus syndrome). When exam results are normal, the history may lead to food allergy as a possible cause. Pharyngeal muscle spasm is undetectable on examination, as is mucosal irritation that causes itching and throat clearing. Irritation and choking following the ingestion of a food can be an immediate or delayed reaction (Table 4–11).

Urticaria and angioedema patients usually present after the episode has resolved with the history that the lips, tongue, and throat had been involved.[51] Food allergy is often involved, and it may be delayed rather than the usually suspected IgE-mediated type.

A "sore throat" reported by a patient usually shows few findings to the physician. A common cause of sore throat without fever is allergy, and yet antibiotics are prescribed repeatedly by many physicians. A proper allergy history may lead to the correct diagnosis. When symptoms continue, the possibility of a viral infection is less likely.

Larynx

Allergy is one of the many causes of hoarseness.[52] Both immediate and delayed forms of allergy may be involved, particularly with foods. The immediate causes are IgE-mediated. History and testing are less difficult when an immediate food reaction is suspected. The delayed forms of allergy, primarily cyclic food allergy, may go unnoticed by the patient and the physician because of the lack of cause-and-effect relationship of ingestion and delayed symptoms. Although laryngologists have mentioned allergy for many years, little has been taught about recognizing delayed food allergy.

Table 4–11   Food-Related Allergic Responses—Mouth and Throat

SYMPTOMS	SIGNS
Oral pain	Perioral rash
Oral itching	Aphthous ulcers
Sore throat (without fever)	Fissures of mouth
Irritation	Throat clearing
Postnasal drip	Swelling
Choking	Dysphagia
Sensation of lump in throat	Angioedema of the lips, tongue, uvula,
Throat clearing	palate and larynx
Clicking	Clicking (uvula striking posterior
Itching roof of mouth or pharynx	pharynx 2° to recurrent clonic
Mouth ulcers	spasms confirmed by stroboscopic
Cold sores	view)

Traditional workups, which test only for immediate allergies, are of little help when delayed allergy is the primary cause of the problem.

Many patients use their voice in their profession and thus qualify as "professional speakers." Intermittent dysphonia is a very significant problem to a schoolteacher, realtor, or salesman, just as it is to a professional singer. When vocal folds look fairly normal on indirect laryngoscopy, and still quite good on fiberoptic laryngoscopy, nonspecific recommendations of voice rest, decongestants, mucolytics, and voice exercises may not eliminate the problem.

Strobovideolaryngoscopy with freeze frame-by-frame study may be very revealing about irregular glottic edge edema and increased, thickened mucus, suggesting delayed food allergy as a possible cause. A proper history, appropriate tests, and subsequent dietary eliminations will often eliminate the symptoms and restore the patient's ability to communicate as well as his or her ability to earn income. A study has been completed using strobovideolaryngoscopy and provocation food tests showing definite changes in the vocal folds (Table 4–12).[53]

Loss of voice is not always psychosomatic even with fairly normal-appearing vocal folds on indirect laryngoscopy. In patients with food allergy, eliminating the offending food can restore the voice.[21]

Lower Respiratory Tract

Nonproductive coughing may be a symptom of food allergy. Except for gastrointestinal gas, this symptom is possibly seen more often than any other.[12] Diagnosing the cause is often difficult, but a 2-week trial on a caveman diet is simple and often very revealing (Table 4–5). If symptoms are at least

Table 4–12   Food-Related Allergic Responses—Larynx

SYMPTOMS	SIGNS
Clearing the throat	Hoarseness or dysphonia
Cough	Edema of vocal folds
Hoarseness	Irregular glottic edge edema seen on freeze-
intermittent	frame study on stroboscopy
constant	Vascular injection of vocal folds
Loss of voice	Polypoid swelling of vocal folds
intermittent	Increased subglottic pressure required to
constant	initiate phonation
Difficulty in initiating phonation	Increased subglottic pressure required to
Difficulty in sustaining phonation	sustain phonation
	Breathiness
	Running out of air too soon in vocalizing
	Increased mucus on vocal folds
	Thick mucus on vocal folds
	Stridor (with angioedema)
	inspiratory if mild to moderate
	inspiratory and expiratory if severe

50% better, specific testing can be undertaken. As with other symptoms of food allergy, good medicine dictates an appropriate workup for cough because some causes are extremely serious (Table 4–13). When complete ENT exam including mirror exams, plus chest exam and chest x-ray, are all negative and an allergy history is positive, appropriate tests may be diagnostic. A food history and food tests may be very important.

Wheezing and Asthma

It has been shown that wheezing in asthma patients can be induced and actually made worse by the ingestion of certain foods such as milk, corn, and wheat.[54] One reason so many patients with asthma do poorly on immunotherapy is that the bronchospasm may be more related to delayed food allergy. The symptoms in a large percentage of asthma patients are significantly improved when delayed food allergy is considered and diagnosed, and the offending foods are eliminated. Immunotherapy for inhalant allergies, control of chemical sensitivities, and other environmental control measures are also important.

Central Nervous System

Personality and behavior changes are often noted by parents when their children ingest particular foods. Children may become hyperactive, lethargic, and even fall asleep after tests to certain foods. Because young children's diets are usually high in dairy and grain products, these are the most common offenders (Table 4–14). When such changes occur in adults, foods are less often suspected because of masking and delay of symptoms. A thorough food allergy history may point to this possibility.

There is considerable controversy about food allergy affecting the central nervous system. Traditional allergists who have studied only IgE mechanisms have published many articles refuting any relationship.[55]

However, there is a large body of literature supporting this relationship.[56–58] Food sensitivity, when involved, is delayed, difficult to study, and difficult to reproduce. There are 223 references in these sources alone indicating the clinical relevance of this subject. There are indeed many more answers needed.

Table 4–13 Food-Related Allergic Responses—Lower Respiratory Tract

SYMPTOMS	SIGNS
Dry cough	Nonproductive cough
Wheezing	Wheezing
Shortness of breath	Shortness of breath

Table 4–14   Food-Related Allergic Responses—Central Nervous System

SYMPTOMS	SIGNS
Hyperactivity	Hyperactivity
Confusion	Confusion
Memory loss	Memory loss
Personality change	Behavior change
Slow mentation	depression
	crying
	mood swings
	Memory loss
	Reduced speed with consecutive arithmetic calculations

Headaches

Migraine headaches may be triggered by food allergy[59,60] and may even be cured by elimination of an offending food. This is certainly preferable to analgesic shots, ergotamine, or sumatriptan (Table 4–15). Every migraine patient deserves a thorough allergy history for both inhalants and foods and possibly a trial on a caveman diet. When an allergic trigger is found, control is very gratifying.

Results of trials with sodium cromoglycate and ketotifen support the view from clinical observation that most cases of migraine are due to food allergy.[61,62]

Sinus headaches: See Sinuses,

Cervical muscle headaches may also be triggered by delayed food allergy. This was an interesting finding to the author when the results of an IgG food test study were tabulated.[12] A surprising number of patients with food allergy who had typical posterior muscle contraction headaches were significantly improved; this caused a shift in traditional thinking—away

Table 4–15   Food-Related Allergic Responses—Headaches

SYMPTOMS	SIGNS
Frontal headaches with upper neck pain	Tightness and pain on palpation of upper cervical musculature with cervical headaches
Temple headaches	Tightness and pain on palpation of temporalis muscle in temporal headaches
Tight band headaches	
Sinus headaches	
Pounding unilateral or bilateral headaches	"Headache facies" with droopy eyes, depressed appearance, holding still
Retro-orbital headaches	Unilateral tearing with Horton's histamine cephalgia
Aura with spots, macular vision, and/or momentary hemianopsia or blindness	

Table 4–16 Food-Related Allergic Responses—Muscular

SYMPTOMS	SIGNS
Tightness	Tightness
Swelling	Swelling
Pain	Spasms
Jerking	Clonic or tonic
Twitching	contractions
Spasms	

from stress, pinched nerves, and supratentorial causes—in those headache patients with positive food allergy histories (see muscle spasm).

Muscular

Muscle spasm can occur anywhere in the body. Several areas have already been mentioned, including posterior cervical (tension) headaches, which may be cleared with elimination of a food (in patients with a positive food allergy history). Clicking in the ear can be caused by stapedial muscle spasm (documented on impedance studies), and clicking in the throat can be clonic uvular muscle spasms. Bladder spasms and enuresis can be related to food allergy (Table 4–16). Even leg cramps may be associated with a food in certain cases. Skeletal muscle appears to be the shock organ in such individuals.[63]

Joints

Rheumatoid arthritis has been studied extensively and certain patients have been shown to have food allergy, with improvement on elimination of the suspected substance.[64,65] Hypersensitivity to milk has been confirmed with a symptom-free period while on a chemically defined antigen-free diet (Vivonex or Tolorex), and reexacerbation with reintroduction of milk.[66] Whereas most rheumatic patients have no allergic diathesis, it is hypothesized that a "delayed" hypersensitivity mechanism, probably not IgE-mediated, may play a role in the food hypersensitivity of these occasional rheumatic disease patients (Table 4–17).[67]

Table 4–17 Food-Related Allergic Responses—Joints

SYMPTOMS	SIGNS
Pain	Redness
Swelling	Swelling
Heat	Increased skin temperature over joint
Decreased or absent ability to function	Limitation of motion
	Subluxation of joints
	Decreased or absent function

Table 4–18   Food Related Allergic Responses—Miscellaneous

SYMPTOMS	SIGNS
Swelling fingers, eyelids, lips, ankles	Edema Fluctuation in weight Inability to remove ring Facial/eyelid edema
Chronic fatigue	Inability to carry out all normal activities due to fatigue
Chills	Chills

Cardiovascular

Arrhythmias have been associated with food sensitivity in certain cases.[68] Tachycardia, angina, myocardial infarction, extrasystoles, and atrial and ventricular fibrillation have also been reported. Nontraumatic phlebitis and vasculitis have also been reported to be triggered by foods.[69]

Miscellaneous

Fluid retention or edema is the hallmark of food allergy in any organ system. When edema is generalized, fluctuation in weight occurs, often as much as 2–5 pounds in a week (Table 4–18).

References

1. Trevino RJ. Food allergies and hypersensitivities. In *The Sinuses,* Donald PJ, Gluckman JL, Rice DH, eds. New York, Raven Press, 1995.
2. Saalman R, Carlsson B, Fallstrom SP, Hanson LA, Ahlstedt S. Antibody dependent cell-mediated cytotoxicity to B-lactoglobulin coated cells with sera from children with cow's milk protein allergy. *Clin Exp Immunol* 1991;85:446–452.
3. Marsh MN. Gluten, major histocompatibility complex, and the small intestine: a molecular and immunobiologic approach to the spectrum of gluten-sensitivity ("celiac sprue"). *Gastroenterology* 1987;102:283–304.
4. DeRitis G, Auricchio S, Jones HW, Lew E, Bernardin JE, Kasarda DD. In-vitro (organ culture) studies of the toxicity of specific A-gliadin peptides in coeliac disease. *Gastroenterology* 1988;94:41–49.
5. Rinkel HJ, Randolph TG, Zeller M. *Food Allergy.* Springfield, IL, Charles C. Thomas: 1951;19.
6. Rinkel HJ, Randolph TG, Zeller M. *Food Allergy,* Springfield, IL, Charles C. Thomas; 1951;12.
7. Brostoff J. *Mechanisms: an Introduction in Food Allergy and Intolerance.* London: Bailliere Tindall; 1987;437–443.
8. Sampson HS. *Food allergy* (review). *J Allergy Clin Immunol* 1989;84:1062–1067.
9. Sachs MI, Yunginger JW. Food induced anaphylaxis. *Immunology Allergy Clin North Am* 1991;11:743–755.
10. Dixon HS, Dixon BJ. Technique of skin endpoint titration. In Mabry RL, ed. *Skin Endpoint Titration.* AAOA Monograph Series. New York: Thieme; 1994;32–36.
11. Crook WG. The Yeast Connection. Jackson, TN: Professional Books; 1995;45–52.

12. Dixon HS. The treatment of delayed food allergy based on specific IgG testing. Submitted to *ENT J* 1997.
13. Bock SA. Prospective appraisal of complaints of adverse reactions to foods in children during the first 3 years of life. *Pediatr London* 1987;79:683–688.
14. Brostoff J. Atopic eczema. In *Food Allergy and Intolerance*. London: Bailliere Tindall; 1987;583.
15. Strobel S. Mechanisms of tolerance and sensitization in the intestine and other organs of the body. *Allergy* 1995; 50 (suppl 20):18–25.
16. Blalock WK. Atopic dermatitis: diagnosis and pathobiology. *J Allergy Clin Immunol* 1976;57:62–79.
17. Williams RI. The Management of Clinical Allergy. Cheyenne, WY: Frontier Printing, 1983;80–86.
18. Winston GB, Lewis CW. Contact urticaria. *Int J Dermatol* 1982;21:573–578.
19. Fisher AA. Contact urticaria from handling meats and fowl. *Cutis* 1982;30:726–729.
20. Champion RH, Robert SO, Carpenter RG, Roger JH. Urticaria and angioedema: a review of 554 patients. *Br J Dermatol* 1969;81:588–597.
21. Author's personal experience.
22. Dougherty TF, Dolowitz DA. Physiologic actions of heparin not related to blood clotting. *Am J Cardiol* 1964;14:18–24.
23. Bonini SE, Bonini ST. The eye. In Mechanisms in Adverse Reactions to Foods. *Allergy* 1995;50 (suppl 20):69–73.
24. Klein JO. Current issues in upper respiratory tract infections in infants and children: rationale for antibacterial therapy. *Pediatr Infec Dis J* 1994;13:5–8.
25. Bernstein JM. The role of IgE-mediated hypersensitivity in the development of otitis media with effusion. *Otolaryngol Clin North Am* 1992;25:197–211.
26. Viscomi GJ. The relationship between allergy and otitis media. In *Otolaryngic Allergy*. King HC, ed. North-Holland, New York. 1981;409–424.
27. Draper WL. Secretory otitis media in children, a study of 540 children. *Laryngoscope* 1967;77:636–653.
28. Mattucci KF, Greenfield BJ. Middle Ear Effusion–Allergy Relationships. *ENT J* 1995;74:752–758.
29. Derebery MJ, Berliner K. Allergic aspects of tinnitus. In Reich JE, ed., *Proceedings of the 5th International Symposium on Tinnitus*, Portland OR, 1995;477–484.
30. Derebery MJ, Valenzuela S. Meniere's syndrome and allergy. *Otolaryngol Clin North Am* 1992;25:213–224.
31. Krause HF. Diagnostic patterns of otolaryngic allergy: symptoms. In *Otolaryngologic Allergy and Immunology*. Philadelphia: WB Saunders, 1989;53.
32. Derebery MJ. Meniere's disease: an immune-complex mediated illness. *Laryngoscope* 1991;101:225–229.
33. Derebery MJ. Allergic and immunologic aspects of Meniere's disease. *Otolaryngol Head Neck Surg*, 1996;114:360–365.
34. Calenoff E, et al. Patients with Meniere's disease possess IgE reacting with herpes family viruses. *Arch Otolaryngol Head Neck Surg* 1995;121:861.
35. Shambaugh GE Jr, Wiet RJ. The endolymphatic sac and Meniere's disease. *Otolaryngol Clin North Am* 1980;13:585.
36. Hill DJ, et al. Manifestations of milk allergy in infancy: clinical and immunological findings. *J Pediatr* 1986;109:270–276.
37. Goldman AS, et al. Milk allergy I, oral challange with milk and isolated milk proteins in allergic children. *Pediatrics* 1963;32:425–443.
38. Bock SA, et al. Studies of hypersensitivity reactions to foods in infants and children. *J Allergy Clin Immunol* 1978;62:327–334.
39. Bindslev-Jensen C. Food Allergy and Intolerance. In Mygind N, Naclerio RM, eds. *Allergy and Non-Allergic Rhinitis, Clinical Aspects*. Copenhagen: Munksgaard 1993;46–50.
40. Stammberger H. Secretion Transport. In *Functional Endoscopic Sinus Surgery*. Philadelphia: BC Decker, 1991;19.
41. Dixon HS, Dixon BJ. Otolaryngic allergy. In *Common Problems of the Head and Neck Region*. Crumley RL, ed. Philadelphia: WB Saunders, 1993;9–23.
42. Williams RI. The Management of Clinical Allergy. Cheyenne, WY: Frontier Printing; 1983;95–97.
43. Pelikan Z. Rhinitis and secretory otitis media: a possible role of food allergy. In Brostoff J, Challacombe SJ, eds. *Food Allergy and Intolerance,* London: Bailliere, Tindall; 1987;468.

44. Downey R III, Parkin RM, MacQuarrie J. Upper airway resistance syndrome: sick, symptomatic but underrecognized. *Sleep* 1993;16:620–623.
45. Partinen M, Jamieson A, Guilleminault C. Long-term outcome for obstructive sleep apnea syndrome patients: mortality. *Chest* 1988;94:1200–1204.
46. Freier S. Sudden infant death syndrome. In *Paedriatric Gastrointestinal Allergy. Clin Allergy* (suppl) 1993;3:597.
47. Cook PR, Nishioka GJ. Allergic rhinosinusitis in the pediatric population. *Otolaryngol Clin North Am* 1996;29:39–56.
48. Knops JL, McCaffrey TV, Kern EB. Physiology, clinical applications. In *Inflammatory Diseases of the Sinuses. Otolaryngol Clin North Am* 1993;26:517–534.
49. Stammberger H. *Functional endoscopic sinus surgery.* Philadelphia: BC Decker, 1991;447–451.
50. Enberg RN. Food-induced oropharyngeal symptoms: the oral allergy syndrome. *Immunol Allergy Clin North Am* 1991;11:767–772.
51. Challacomb SJ. Oral manifestations of food allergy and intolerance. In Brostoff J, Challacombe SJ, eds., *Food Allergy and Intolerance.* London: Bailliere and Tindall; 1987;511–520.
52. Dixon HS. Allergy and laryngeal disease. *Otolaryngol Clin North Am* 1992;25:239–250.
53. Dixon HS. Dysphonia and delayed food allergy, a provocation/neutralization study with strobovideolaryngoscopy. Submitted to *Otolaryngol Head Neck Surg* 1996.
54. Wraith DG. Asthma. In Brostoff J, Challacombe SJ, eds. *Food Allergy and Intolerance.* London: Bailliere Tindall; 1987;486–497.
55. Anderson JA. The Brain. In *Atlas on Mechanisms in Adverse Reactions to Foods. Allergy* 1995;50 (suppl 20):79–81.
56. Egger J. The hyperkinetic syndrome. In Brostoff J, Challacombe SJ, eds. *Food Allergy and Intolerance.* London: Bailliere Tindall; 1987;674–687.
57. Pearson DJ, Rix KJB. Psychological effects of food allergy. In Brostoff J, Challacombe SJ, eds. *Food Allergy and Intolerance.* London: Bailliere Tindall; 1987;688–708.
58. Bell IR. Effects of food on the central nervous system. In Brostoff J, Challacombe SJ, eds. *Food Allergy and Intolerance.* London: Bailliere Tindall; 1987;709–721.
59. Monro J. Food induced migraine. In Brostoff J, Challacombe SJ, eds. *Food Allergy and Intolerance.* London: Bailliere Tindall; 1987;633–665.
60. Egger J. Food allergy and the central nervous system in childhood. In Brostoff J, Challacombe SJ, eds. *Food Allergy and Intolerance.* London: Bailliere Tindall; 1987;666–673.
61. Monro J, Carini C, Brostoff J. Migraine is a food allergic disease. *Lancet* 1984;2:719–721.
62. Borge P. Ketotifen in multiple allergies. *Res Clin Forums* 1982;4:79–83.
63. Travell JG, Simons DG. *Myofascial Pain and Dysfunction. The Trigger Point Manual.* Baltimore: Williams and Wilkins; 1983;153–154.
64. Parke AL, Hughes GRV. Rheumatoid arthritis and food: a case study. *Br Med J* 1981;282:2027–2029.
65. Hicklin JA, McEwen LM, Morgan JE. The effect of diet in rheumatoid arthritis. *Clin Allergy* 1980;10:463.
66. Panush RS, Stroud RM, Webster EM. Food-induced (allergic) arthritis. Inflammatory arthritis exacerbated by milk. *Arthritis Rheum* 1986;29:220–226.
67. Panush RS, ed. Nutrition and rheumatic diseases. *Rheum Dis Clin* 1991;17:VII–XIV, 197–456.
68. Harkavy J. *Vascular Allergy and Its Systemic Manifestations.* Washington: Butterworths; 1963.
69. Rae WJ, Brown OD. Cardiovascular disease in response to chemicals and foods. In Brostoff J, Challacombe SJ, eds. *Food Allergy and Intolerance.* London: Bailliere Tindall; 1987;737–753.

♦ 5 ♦

The Diagnosis of Food Allergy

HAMILTON S. DIXON, M.D.

The maze of adverse food reactions is so complex that no single test can address all the possibilities. The purpose of this chapter is to present an overview of this subject, but, more specifically, to present the essential material to assist the practitioner in developing a simpler and more straightforward approach to this very confusing subject.

The diagnosis of food allergy has been an almost completely overlooked science. Because of confusion and controversy over testing procedures and consequently treatment protocols, the issue of food allergy is often sidetracked or dismissed completely. Resident physicians receive no training in this field except in IgE-immediate food allergy. This is only a minor part of the food allergy problem. Postgraduate specialists also receive little or no information, thus little appreciation for the diagnosis and treatment of food allergy exists.

The most important part of any diagnosis is a careful and thorough history. In a doctor's office, however, this history is usually confined to the exact problem for which the patient is being seen. For example, if a patient presents with a headache, that problem is addressed and no further history may be taken. If the exam results appear normal, the patient is frequently dismissed with a prescription and asked to return if the problem recurs. Finding the correct cause of the headache obviously requires further history, a complete head and neck examination, and often further workup. If this is still unsuccessful, going back to the history is the next step. This requires a knowledge of the differential diagnosis in order to ask the correct questions. Expensive computed tomography (CT) scans are not necessarily indicated at this point.

Proper history taking will help us recognize two types of immunologic reactions to foods that must be considered separately. Fixed or immediate reactions are IgE-mediated and are often recognized by the patient because there is usually a cause-and-effect relationship. If the patient eats a particular food, he immediately gets sick, breaks out, or has some definite symptoms. He quickly learns that this particular food causes the problem. It always happens every time that same food is ingested. He can easily see a cause-and-effect relationship, and almost always knows which food to eliminate.

Cyclic or delayed food allergy, on the other hand, has no cause-and-effect relationship and is immune complex–mediated with complement activation, related to IgG. It is estimated that only 5% of food allergy is immediate and that 95% is delayed.[1] True anaphylaxis to food is rare, but many other problems can definitely be related to delayed food allergy. Recurrent otitis media in childhood or migraine headaches are quite common and often have delayed food allergy as the underlying cause.

Traditional food allergy texts contain considerable scientific information on IgE-mediated food allergy but fall short in the area of diagnosing delayed food allergy. The double-blind placebo-controlled food challenge is considered the gold standard.[2] This may be effective for immediate food allergy, but not for delayed food allergy. Certain rules must be followed because of the nature of cyclic or delayed food allergy. These rules are not adequately delineated in the "traditional" method,[3] but are critical for successful diagnosis.

The diagnosis of fixed food allergy is well agreed upon, but the concept of cyclic or delayed food allergy is the main area of different viewpoints between the internal medicine–pediatric allergists and the otolaryngic allergists. This clinical "syndrome" was discovered in the late 1930s and 1940s[4,5] and further documented in 1951[6] (Fig. 1–1). This cyclic food allergy concept is now known as *delayed food allergy*. It is thought to be mainly immune complex–mediated with complement activation or type III hypersensitivity. When cyclic food allergy is in the masked stage, symptoms go unrecognized and are delayed with no cause-and-effect relationship. After 4 days of total elimination, the patient is in a hyperacute phase. This unmasks the symptoms, makes them much more obvious, much less delayed (seeming rather immediate at times), and thus the symptoms are easily confused with type I hypersensitivity. This unmasking through elimination is the key to the oral challenge feeding test, the gold standard in food allergy diagnosis.

The traditional criteria for food allergy diagnosis are listed as follows:[7] Major criteria:

1. Class II or higher IgE radioallergosorbent test (RAST)
2. Positive prick test

Minor criteria:

1. History of urticaria or pruritus
2. History of postprandial nausea, diarrhea, or abdominal pain

One major and two minor criteria are required for the diagnosis of food allergy according to this "traditional" point of view. General allergists are just now beginning to recognize this important aspect of delayed food allergy, but it has been noted only in a guest editorial.[8] Knicker states that although classic allergies involving the skin, airway, and digestive tract may and do occur with delayed food reactions, "they may also include a bewildering array of symptoms (well over 200 food-related symptoms and 50 medical conditions at last count) in various organ systems."

The purpose of this chapter is to encompass a much broader overview of food allergy—to include also cyclic or delayed reactions that make up as much as 95% of the overall problem. Thus, diagnostic endeavors must include this aspect of food allergy in order to be successful.

Screening Tests

Food Allergy History

The hallmark of any diagnosis is the history. With many cases of immediate food allergy, the cause-and-effect relationship makes itself known to the patient and history taking is therefore easy. However, with delayed food allergy, normal history taking is not helpful. If the right questions are asked, however, this possibility can be strongly suspected and further testing recommended. A typical food allergy questionnaire is shown in Chapter 4 (Table 4–1). The physician must personally review this questionnaire with the patient, which can be done in 5 minutes. Time must be taken to be sure that symptoms the patient takes for granted as normal are recorded.

Nasal Cytology

Nasal cytology is a simple test, but it must be done correctly.[9] Whereas eosinophils indicate pollen and inhalant allergy, basophils (or tissue mast cells) when seen in nasal secretions signify food allergy.[10] The equipment for this test is simple, and highly trained technicians are not required to do the test. The results can lead to the correct diagnosis.

Elimination Diets

Most physicians use elimination diets by simply eliminating foods and adding them back to the diet one at a time to see if any symptoms occur.[11] This is time-consuming and is generally not a worthwhile endeavor. In order for this test to have any validity, an individual food must be totally eliminated for 2 full weeks to see if the symptoms disappear. It then takes several days back on the food to see if symptoms recur. This would have to be repeated at least three times to be certain of the cause-and-effect relationship. If 15 foods were to be investigated, 45 weeks might be required. It is impractical for a patient to keep adequate food and symptom diaries for that long. However, highly suspect foods—such as cow's milk in a baby's diet—may be eliminated with excellent results, requiring no further testing.

Caveman Diet

This primitive diet is an excellent screening test for food allergy and is very cost effective. It is simply a diet limited to fresh fruits and vegetables, and boiled or broiled meat, for 2 weeks. The only beverages allowed are fruit juice, vegetable juice, and water. This gets out of the diet the most frequent food offenders, typically corn, egg, wheat, milk, soy, and peanut. The immune complexes and food antigens are metabolized and excreted within the 2-week period, and if food intolerance is a big part of the patient's problem, symptoms will be significantly better. At least 50% improvement in 2 weeks should be seen before one recommends specific testing (See Chapter 4, Table 4–5, for details of this diet.)

Chemically Defined Diet

This is an excellent way to screen for food allergy or intolerance by replacing food with a chemically defined diet (Vivonex or Tolorex*). The diet is devoid of all food antigens and is nutritionally sound. All ingredients are in digested form and can be assimilated through the gastric mucosa. With no fecal residue, this diet gives the gut a rest and completely avoids the assimilation of the macromolecules responsible for site attachment of immune complexes at the shock organ. A 2-week trial answers the question as to whether the patient's symptoms are due to food intolerance. It also convinces the patient that further testing is needed (Appendix 5–1).[12]

Diet Diary Computer Analysis

This is a new concept that requires extremely careful documentation by the patient of all ingredients of every food eaten including all condiments, which is very difficult when dining out. All symptoms must be recorded in detail at the time of onset and disappearance. This information is then entered into a complex computer program for analysis with the expectation that offending foods can be identified without in vivo or in vitro testing.[13]

In Vivo Food Tests

Oral Challenge Feeding Test

At first look, the double-blind, placebo-controlled food challenge would appear to be the best test.[2] However, there are a number of problems with this approach that have kept it as a research tool.

* Sandoz Nutritional Corp., Minneapolis, MN.

1. Only a limited number of foods are available in the freeze-dried form.
2. After the capsule dissolves in the stomach, eructation may allow identification of the food, particularly those with a strong flavor.
3. It is difficult to hide the strong taste, color, or odor of a large quantity of a food in a liquid vehicle.
4. There is a good chance of a bias for both the patient and examiner because a placebo is expected following a previous positive test. Multiple tests in random fashion are recommended but are admittedly impractical (the otolaryngic method recommends only one challenge test at a time, waiting one week between tests—a concept very different from multiple challenges in one sitting).
5. Freeze-dried foods are changed and their antigenicity may be altered.
6. The route of exposure is changed, removing olfaction, bronchial inhalation, and pharyngeal contact.
7. The provoking dose of a freeze-dried food may vary from the natural form. Data on weight equivalents is limited.

The "open" oral challenge feeding test is also not perfect. Problems include the following:

1. A positive test does not indicate the underlying mechanism involved.
2. The selection of foods to be tested depends on the diligent use of screening procedures, such as medical history, food and symptom diaries, trials of elimination diets, skin testing, and in vitro tests.
3. Associated factors may not be duplicated, such as postprandial exercise-induced allergic reactions, combinations of foods, inhalants, hormonal changes, gastrointestinal disturbances, intercurrent illnesses, or emotional stress.[3]

Despite these problems, the challenge feeding test is the most reliable, but only if the rules are strictly followed.[14] Because it takes only 4 days for the food antigens and their immune complexes to be metabolized following total elimination, this converts the masked phase of food allergy to the hyperacute phase.[15] The food challenge is then done on the fifth day. When a large amount of the pure food is ingested after 4 days of total elimination, a large amount of antigen is suddenly ingested, which forms a great many immune complexes. This increased number of antigen–antibody complexes stimulates the complement system and results in signs and symptoms that are magnified compared to those to which the patient is accustomed. This fifth-day window of opportunity extends for a few days but wanes, and the effectiveness of the test diminishes gradually. If the challenge is done with incomplete elimination, the hyperacute phase will not be attained and an offending food will not be discovered.

The hidden foods are the most common offenders. These include milk, corn, egg, wheat, soy, and peanut, and it takes considerable coaching to educate a patient on how to totally eliminate these foods from the diet.

Regarding delayed food allergy, this same 4-day concept is the basis of the rotary-diversified diet, which states that one would not become allergic to new foods if ingested only every fourth day.[16] This same concept is also the basis of selecting foods to be tested. If one does not become allergic to a food unless it is eaten at least every third day, then the only foods that need be tested are those eaten twice weekly or more. Delayed allergic sensitivity depends on frequency of ingestion as well as amount. Thus foods eaten most frequently are tested first. Frequent ingestion may constitute food addiction in some patients and may lead to markedly uncomfortable withdrawal symptoms during this 4-day elimination period.[17]

INSTRUCTIONS FOR ORAL CHALLENGE FEEDING TEST

1. Complete a 2-week diet diary. This must include all condiments and spices as well as brands of prepared foods, including brands of fast foods at restaurants. Select only those foods eaten twice weekly or more. Start with the most frequently eaten food.
2. Totally eliminate the test food for 4 days.
3. Eat an early breakfast, still omitting the food to be tested. Nothing—including food, beverages, or medications—should be taken after breakfast until the test is done. Smoking should be avoided.
4. Prepare the food to be tested according to the instructions (Appendix 5–2).
5. Arrive at the office 30 minutes in advance to allow for a quiet time. No loud talking, laughing, or noise during the test.
6. Eat the first quantity of the test food within a 5-minute period.
7. If there are no recognizable symptoms within 1 hour, a second portion the size of the first is eaten.
8. Record all signs and symptoms as follows:
   a. List all signs and symptoms that are present prior to the food challenge (patients often need help, for they may not recognize "symptoms" that are always present).
   b. List all additional signs and symptoms every 5 minutes during the first hour.
   c. List additional signs and symptoms every 15 minutes during the second hour.
   d. Delayed symptoms or reactions can occur up to 18 hours after ingestion. Record all signs and symptoms at home and call the office to report these the following day.
   e. Record all signs and symptoms such as sniffing, sneezing, blowing, coughing, itching, headache, fatigue, GI symptoms, change in pulse, and so on.
9. Severe symptoms may be relieved by taking Alka-Seltzer Gold, unflavored milk of magnesia, or high doses of vitamin C or by breathing oxygen after the test is completed. Oral cromolyn sodium may also be helpful.

10. This test may be done at home provided there is no history of severe reactions and the patient is not asthmatic and is well instructed.
11. Any cooked food is prepared at home and warmed at the office.
12. Two foods cannot be accurately tested on the same day. Only one food per week is recommended.
13. Canned or frozen food can be used if no sugar, filler, or preservatives have been added.
14. All foods must be pure. Fresh is best.
15. Do *not* test for any known food allergy.

Prick Test

Like scratch tests, these tests elicit too many false-positive and false-negative responses, with poor specificity.[18] Yet this is the preferred food test done by internal medicine–pediatric allergists.[19]

Intradermal Provocative Food Test

The intradermal provocative food test (IPFT) was conceived by Rinkel[6] and further developed by Lee.[20] Its use has remained limited by a relatively small number of physicians in otolaryngic allergy and environmental medicine and has never gained acceptance by internal medicine–pediatric allergists.[21] There are numerous published double-blind studies confirming the efficacy of this test.[22] The most definitive work is the triple-blind, crossover, placebo-controlled, multicenter provocation-neutralization study by King and colleagues.[23]

The IPFT is simply a skin test that depends on a potent dose of the extract rather than the dilute doses used in inhalant testing. It is therefore dangerous in the case of a serious IgE-mediated food sensitivity, particularly in a brittle asthmatic. Three rules must preface the use of this test:

1. Never test a patient for a food that historically has produced a severe reaction. If the patient is quite sure of a specific sensitivity, the reaction is most likely IgE-mediated and is easy to confirm by IgE RAST.
2. Test only for foods that are in the diet on a regular basis. Foods must be eaten twice weekly or more to develop any significant delayed reaction.
3. Do not test exquisitely sensitive patients or patients who are taking high doses of steroids, such as brittle asthmatics. Asthmatics who are not taking steroids may also be at risk, and testing should be considered only by trained clinicians experienced in dealing with status asthmaticus and prepared for severe reactions.

Because a potent dose of extract is needed to elicit a response in delayed allergy, provocation of signs and symptoms often occurs, just as it does with inhalant testing if too large a dose is used.

Fivefold dilutions of extracts are used, such as they are with skin endpoint titration,[24] vial testing following modified RAST, and mixing testing and treatment sets for inhalants.

This test is not recommended for the untrained physician. The American Academy of Otolaryngic Allergy (AAOA)* Foundation conducts basic and advanced courses in otolaryngic allergy. Instruction courses are conducted at the AAOA annual meeting held in conjunction with the American Academy of Otolaryngology–Head and Neck Surgery Annual Meeting, all under the aegis of the American Board of Otolaryngology. A variety of other standalone courses teaching these techniques are available and made known through the AAOA office. It is advisable to visit an AAOA fellow for on-site training in this test.

For the IPFT, with other skin tests, antihistamines must be stopped for several days in advance.

INSTRUCTIONS FOR INTRADERMAL PROVOCATIVE/
NEUTRALIZATION FOOD TEST

1. A diet diary should be accurately and completely filled out for 2 weeks in order to select all foods that are consumed twice per week or more. These foods are then arranged in order of frequency of ingestion.
2. The food must be consumed on a regular basis. If the patient has been on some kind of elimination diet as a trial, this must be terminated. The minimum time to reestablish regular consumption and thus masked or delayed allergy is 2 weeks. This fact is unknown to those physicians who consider that the validity of this test, like any other, is confirmed by its repeatability. When this test is repeated the next day and a negative response is obtained, its validity is incorrectly questioned.[11] A positive provocative food test should not be repeated for at least 2 weeks, until sensitivity is reestablished through regular consumption.
3. Because a potent dose of extract is needed to elicit a response in delayed allergy, provocation of symptoms often occurs, just as it does with inhalant testing if too large a dose is used.
4. The patient is asked to report on any symptoms that were present at the start of the test, and these are recorded on the test sheet.
5. A negative control is applied by placing 0.05 cm^3 of a no. 1 dilution (1:100) of glycerin intradermally. This is done because all extracts are made with 50% glycerin, a preservative used to maintain potency for shelf life; 0.05 cm^3 creates a 7 mm wheal. The wheal size in 10 minutes is recorded on the IPFT form (Appendix 5–3).
6. This test is done in single-blind fashion—that is, the patient is unaware of which food is being applied.

---

* American Academy of Otolaryngic Allergy, 8455 Colesville Road, Suite 745, Silver Springs, MD 20910-9998

7. 0.05 cm³ of the no. 1 dilution (1:100) of the test food extract is applied intradermally. This creates a 7 mm wheal.
8. The wheal size is measured and recorded on the IPFT form in 10 minutes.
9. The test is considered negative if the wheal growth is the same as or less than the negative glycerin control within 10 minutes.
10. The test is considered positive if the wheal grows 2 mm more than the negative glycerin control wheal within 10 minutes.
11. Careful clinical observation by an experienced professional is required for signs of a provoked reaction. These signs are recorded on the IPFT form on the appropriate time line. A review of the many possible signs listed in Chapter 4 is recommended for study.
12. The patient is asked to report any symptoms that have occurred since the onset of the test. These are documented on the IPFT form on the correct time line. Similarly, the symptoms of food allergy listed in Chapter 4 are recommended for study.
13. The skin response is more important than provoked symptoms.[23]
14. Once a positive wheal is recorded, it is advisable to neutralize that wheal as well as neutralizing any provoked symptoms. Neutralization stops the allergic reaction, makes the positive wheal disappear, reverses any symptoms produced, and determines a treatment dose for immunotherapy. The neutralizing dose always results in a negative wheal. The original positive wheal simultaneously reverts to a negative wheal.
15. To find the neutralizing dose, 0.05 cm³ of the next weaker dilution (no. 2 dilution or 1:500) is applied intradermally. This test is also read and recorded in 10 minutes. If this is still a reacting wheal (ie, 2 mm larger than the negative glycerin control), the provoked symptoms are still present, and the original positive wheal is still positive, then this is not the neutralizing dose.
16. The next weaker dilution is then applied, i.e., 0.05 cm³ of the no. 3 dilution (1:2500) intradermally. If the provoked symptoms stop or are reversed, this new wheal remains negative, and the original positive wheal disappears, then this no. 3 dilution is determined to be the neutralizing dose.
17. Testing is terminated once a positive test occurs and neutralization is complete.
18. If testing is negative, one may proceed to test another food.
19. If a significant systemic reaction occurs, attempting to neutralize the reaction can be done, but this may not be possible and instituting established emergency measures is of prime importance.
20. If neutralization cannot be achieved and symptoms are not serious, standard pharmacotherapy suffices, along with careful follow-up.
21. The neutralizing dose is the strongest dilution that results in a negative wheal.

This same mechanism can be used when a "flash" response occurs with

Table 5–1 Efficacy of the Intradermal Provocative Food Test[23]

TEST	SENSITIVITY	SPECIFICITY	EFFICIENCY
IPFT Skin Response	79.7%	72.4%	76.8%
IPFT Provocation of Symptoms	59.6%	92.1%	73.0%

skin end-point titration inhalant testing (Table 5–1). Progressive whealing leads to the sudden occurrence of a 15 mm or greater wheal with pseudopodia, erythema, itching, and provoked symptoms. The neutralizing dose will stop these provoked symptoms and make the large "flash" wheal disappear. The neutralizing dose is almost always one dilution weaker (one five-fold dilution weaker) and becomes the end point. This end point of reaction becomes the beginning point of immunotherapy for inhalants from which doses are escalated to the maximum tolerated dose. With delayed food allergy, however, the neutralizing dose is not escalated. This represents another major difference in viewpoint between the internal medicine–pediatric allergists and otolaryngic allergists. The mechanism of neutralization has been proposed by Trevino.[15]

Dimsoft Test

This test combines lyophilized food extract with dimethyl sulfoxide and is applied as a patch test. Thus, non-water-soluble food extract is carried through the skin to react with underlying tissues.[25] Though this test did receive FDA approval, too many false-positive reactions have kept it from general use.

In Vitro Food Tests

IgE RAST

When food sensitivity manifests as an immediate reaction, this test is a simple and effective tool.[26] Because it is an in vitro test, it is free from danger.

The patient's history is the best determinant to decide whether this test is indicated. There is not uniform agreement as to whether a few foods should be included in a standard RAST panel for pollens and inhalants. Some patients, mainly those with multiple high sensitivities to inhalants and a high total IgE, will show positive IgE to hidden foods that were not suspected by history. This author does not count foods positive by IgE unless they are a class II or higher. Removing these foods from the diet is helpful to reduce the total allergic load. After IgE-positive foods are eliminated, the patient can often see relief of symptoms and is then more willing to omit those foods.

This test is most useful when a patient has a positive history of an immediate food reaction, especially anaphylaxis, and specific documentation is urgent.

Immune Complex Food Test

Most efforts at food diagnosis involve looking for cyclic or delayed offenders (hidden food allergy); because this is mostly a type III immune complex–mediated phenomenon, testing for immune complexes makes sense. Measuring immune complex levels has remained experimental because of high cost, the limited number of foods available, and the small number of laboratories qualified to do this test.[27]

IgG RAST

Correlation between immune complex levels and IgG levels is not perfect, but measuring specific IgG for foods is a standard RAST procedure. IgG foods is considered a screening procedure because elevated levels do not necessarily confirm a cause-and-effect relationship; that is, a high level for wheat does not prove that wheat is causing the patient's symptoms. If this test is used, an experienced clinician must take these results in combination with a detailed history and proceed to individual oral challenge tests to establish the cause-and-effect relationship.

It has been the author's experience that only the most obsessive-compulsive patients have been willing to complete a battery of challenge tests, either in the office or on their own at home despite the test's accuracy and cost effectiveness. Likewise the average patient has not been willing to return again and again to complete all the intradermal provocative tests necessary to recommend a proper elimination and substitution diet. This led to revisiting the imperfect IgG test for foods. One hundred twenty-five patients were identified by history as very likely to have food allergy, and IgG tests were done. No attempt was made to prove cause-and-effect relationship by oral challenge, but only to eliminate all positive-test foods for 6 months. Significant improvement in symptoms occurred within 2 weeks, confirming the value of this approach. Careful follow-up was obtained on 80 patients. Special value was obtained in 11 patients who had entirely negative IgE RAST for inhalants. It is very disconcerting to obtain a very positive allergy history from a patient and then get an entirely negative RAST and/or skin test. Interestingly, this group of 11 patients uniformly had significantly positive food allergy histories, and subsequently positive results were found on IgG food testing. These results were confirmed when those patients uniformly cleared their symptom complex when the positive foods were eliminated.

Likewise, special value was also obtained in the 20 patients with debilitating symptoms who also obtained remarkable improvement after elimination of positive IgG foods.

Considering only those patients who obtained at least 75% or more improvement in symptoms, the overall improvement rate was 71%. Though this is a lower efficacy rate than with IPFT, and considerably lower than oral challenge, patient acceptance has been so much better that the completion of workup rate is far higher. Very few patients have needed or desired to proceed to oral challenge confirmation, and the overall satisfaction rate has improved. Though this study was not done in double-blind research fashion and would therefore be considered anecdotal, the value has been very apparent clinically.[28]

Dockhorn has studied specific IgG foods extensively and finds this test of definite value in treating his patients. After each of his research studies has been presented at the American Academy of Allergy and Immunology, its official journal, the *Journal of Allergy and Clinical Immunology*, has refused to publish his work, always recommending further studies. When these further studies were completed and presented, the same response occurred. Thus his work remains largely unpublished except as abstracts.[29–31]

A few investigators continue to work with IgG foods and find the test of value†‡[32,33] On the other hand, other investigators have studied this subject and have concluded that the predictive value of the test is too low to recommend it for routine use.[34] Thus, this remains a controversial subject needing more study. One stumbling block is that normal subjects can have IgG levels to specific foods, with no symptoms.[31] This may not be any different from normal subjects who have positive skin tests or RAST tests with no symptoms of inhalant allergy.

Still others have recommended doing both specific IgE and IgG or IgG$_4$ for foods. This does have a better predictive value but has a higher cost. Using specific IgG$_4$ rather than specific IgG for foods represents another unresolved area. Nalebuff states that the range of results in IgE RAST from the least to the most positive represents an increase of 80 times, whereas IgG RAST for foods has only a sixfold increase. IgG$_4$, on the other hand, has the same 80-fold increase as IgE. Others, however, feel this is not a critical issue.‡§

Whether IgG$_4$ has a better predictive value than IgG for foods is unresolved. Numerous studies have been done[35–37] with a thorough review by Shakib.[38] Harris, Bellanti, and colleagues showed that either IgE or IgG$_4$ had a predictive value of 71% for those patients who tested positive by blinded food challenges; when both tests were done together, the agreement rose to 91%.[39]

† Nalebuff DJ, personal communication
‡ Braly J, personal communication
§ Harris NS, personal communication.

Cytotoxic Food Test

This test was first introduced by Black,[40] refined by Bryan and Bryan,[41] and further advocated by Boyles.[42] It combines the patient's white cells with a food antigen, and resultant morphologic changes are studied. Because of technical difficulties in performing the test accurately, its reproducibility was poor and the FDA disapproved its use. When properly done, however the cytotoxic test did have merit.[43]

ALCAT Test

This test is a newer version of the cytotoxic food test, with wider parameters and better technology.[44] It has gained little acceptance in the United States but is used in Europe.

Lymphocyte Transformation Test

This is another newer technique measuring lymphocyte morphologic changes. Its hope for the future is that clinical comparisons will verify its validity.[45]

Basophil Histamine Release Test

This test is used for inhalant antigens and may hold promise for foods, even for non–immunologically mediated food reactions. This may expand in vitro testing but would only be applicable when the release of histamine is the mechanism involved.[46,47]

Summary

Though the maze of adverse food reactions is confusing and food intolerance can involve non-immunologic mechanisms, considering an allergic cause first is helpful. Obtaining a food allergy history is not difficult if the correct questions are asked. Deciding on the most appropriate tests is a matter for the physician to determine with the patient. Screening procedures may be considered, but the oral challenge feeding test is the most accurate. In vitro tests followed by oral challenge may be preferred if the patient will agree. Alternative approaches include in vitro tests alone (IgE and/or IgG or IgG$_4$) or the intradermal provocative food test. A variety of other tests are presented.

Because there is still considerable science lacking in our understanding of the various mechanisms of food allergy and intolerance, concomitant allergy, chemical sensitivities, and yeast-connected illness, there is no single test for food allergy that is entirely satisfactory. The likelihood that one test will emerge as the standard is not great because so many different mechanisms are involved. An astute clinician oriented to the possibility—and a knowledgeable staff,¶ to provide patient education and dietary advice—is the best start for food allergy diagnosis.

References

1. Boyles JH Jr. Introduction to food allergy: history and characteristics. In: Krause HF, ed. *Otolaryngic Allergy and Immunology.* Philadelphia: WB Saunders; 1989;218.
2. Bock SA, Sampson HA, Atkins FJ, et al. Double-blind placebo-controlled food challenge (DBPCFC) as an office procedure: a manual. *J Allergy Clin Immunol* 1988;82:986–997.
3. Bahna SL. Practical considerations in food allergy testing. In: Anderson JA, ed. *Food Allergy, Immunol and Allergy Clin North Amer* 1991;11:843–850.
4. Rinkel HJ. Food allergy. *J Kansas Med Soc* 1936;37:177.
5. Rinkel HJ. Food allergy I: The role of food allergy in internal medicine. *Ann Allergy* 1944;2:115.
6. Rinkel HJ, Randolph TG, Zeller M. *Food Allergy.* Springfield, IL: Charles C. Thomas, 1951;19.
7. Sampson H. Adverse reactions to foods. In: Middleton E, et al, eds. *Allergy Principles and Practice.* St. Louis: CV Mosby; 1993;1675–1678.
8. Knicker WT. The spectrum of adverse food reactions in subjects having respiratory allergic disease. *Ann Allergy* 1994;73:282–284.
9. Anderson HA. Practical nasal cytology: key to the problem nose. *J Contin Educ ORL Allergy* 1979;53.
10. Bryan MA. Nasal cytograms in the diagnosis of allergy. *Trans Am Soc Ophthalmol Otolaryngol Allergy* 1967;8:24.
11. Golbert TM. Food allergy and immunologic diseases of the gastrointestinal tract. In: Patterson R, ed. *Allergic Diseases, Diagnosis and Management.* Philadelphia: JB Lippincott; 1985;467–468.
12. Dockhorn RJ, Smith TC. The use of a chemically defined hypoallergenic diet (Vivonex) in the management of patients with suspected food allergy/intolerance. *Ann Allergy* 1981;47:264–266.
13. Kueper TV, Martinelli DL, Konetzki W, Stamerjohn RW, Magill JB. Identification of problem foods using food and symptom diaries. *Otolaryngol Head Neck Surg* 1995;112:415–420.
14. Williams RI. The Specific diagnosis of food allergy. In *The Management of Clinical Allergy.* Cheyenne Wy: Frontier Printing; 1983;119–137.
15. Trevino RJ. Food allergies and hypersensitivities. In: Donald PJ, Gluckman JL, Rice DH eds. *The Sinuses.* New York: Raven Press; 1995;126.
16. King HC. Antigen selection for food allergy testing. In: Krause HF, ed. *Otolaryngic Allergy and Immunology.* Philadelphia: WB Saunders; 1989;242.
17. King HC. Food allergy diagnosis. In: *An Otolaryngologist's Guide to Allergy.* New York: Thieme; 1990:104–119.
18. Fadal RG. Introduction to food allergy and other adverse reactions to foods. *Res Staff Phys* 1988;34:23–33.
19. Atkins FM. Food-induced urticaria. In: Metcalfe DD, Sampson HA, Simon RA, eds. *Food Allergy, Adverse Reactions to Foods and Food Additives.* London: Blackwell Scientific Publications; 1991;132–133.
20. Lee CH, Shepherd EM, Scala LS. Foods. In: *Allergy Neutralization—the Lee Method.* St. Joseph, MO: Tri Sigma Press; 1987;67–88.
21. Jewett DL, Feing D, Greenberg MH. A double-blind study of symptom provocation to Determine Food Sensitivity. *N Engl J Med* 1990;323:429–433.
22. King HC. Double-blind controlled studies of food allergy published in the literature, Appendix 5. In: *An Otolaryngologist's Guide to Allergy.* New York: Thieme; 1990;239.
23. King WP, et al. Provocation-neutralization: a two-part study, Part I, The intracutaneous

¶ Paramedical personnel training is available through the ASOAT, The American Society of Otolaryngic Allergy Technicians, with annual meetings in conjunction with the American Academy of Otolaryngic Allergy.

provocation food test: a multi-center study; Part II, Subcutaneous neutralization therapy: a multi-center study. *Otolaryngol Head Neck Surg* 1988;99:263–277.

24. Dixon HS, Dixon BJ. Technique of skin endpoint titration. In: Mabry RL, ed. *Skin Endpoint Titration.* New York: Thieme; 1994;32–36.
25. Breneman JC, Sweeney M, Robert R. Immunology of delayed-type food allergy. *Immunol Allergy Pract* 1991;13:6.
26. Waikman FJ. Food allergy: a comparative diagnostic study. In: Johnson F, ed. *Allergy: Including IgE in Diagnosis and Treatment.* Miami, Fl: Symposia Specialists; 1979;145–154.
27. Dockhorn RA, Necessary PC, Leary HL Jr, Halsey JF. Allergen-specific immune complexes in food sensitive patients. *Ann Allergy* 1984;52:232.
28. Dixon HS. The treatment of delayed food allergy based on IgG food testing. Submitted to *ENT J* 1997.
29. Dockhorn RJ. Clinical studies of food allergy in infants and children. *Ann Allergy,* 1987; 59 Part II: 137–140.
30. Dockhorn RJ, Frick OL. Delayed-onset food reactions, adverse reactions to foods and additives. Proceedings of the VI International Food Allergy Symposium, 1987.
31. Dockhorn RJ, O'Bryan JJ, Dockhorn DW, Halsey JF. Effect of diet on food IgG responses in healthy non-allergic individuals. *Ann Allergy* 1991;59:104.
32. Hamburger RN, et al. Severe anemic and chronic bronchitis associated with a markedly elevated specific IgG to cow's milk protein. *Ann Allergy* 1985;55:38–40.
33. Hamburger RN, et al. Long-term studies in the prevention of food allergy: patterns of IgG anti-cow's milk antibody responses. *Ann Allergy* 1987;59:175–178.
34. Trevino RJ, Rapoport AS. Problems with in-vitro diagnosis of food allergy. *ENT Journal* 1990;69:42–46.
35. Perelmutter I. IgG_4: Non-IgE-mediated atopic disease. *Ann Allergy* 1984;52:64–68.
36. Halpern GM. Recent Applications of IgG_4 in Diagnosis and Management of Allergic Disease, *Immunol Allergy Practice* 1986;8:386–396.
37. Harris NS, Rock HS, Leese PT. The development of specific IgG_4 after immunotherapy with standardized extracts. *N Engl Regional Allergy Proc* 1987;8:429–435.
38. Shakib F. The role of IgG_4 in food allergy. In: Brostoff J, Challacombe S, eds. *Food Allergy and Intolerance.* London: Bailliere-Tindall; 1987;898–906.
39. El Rafei A, Peters SM, Harris NS, Bellanti JA. Diagnostic value of IgG_4 measurement in patients with food allergy. *Ann Allergy* 1989;62:94–99.
40. Black AB. A New diagnostic method in allergic disease. *Pediatrics* 1956;7:716–724.
41. Bryan WTK, Bryan MA. Cytotoxic reactions in the diagnosis of food allergy. *Otolaryngol Clin North Am* 1971;4:523–533.
42. Boyles JH Jr. The validity of using the cytotoxic food test in clinical allergy. *ENT Journal* 1977;56.
43. Holopainen E, et al. Cytotoxic leukocyte reaction. *Acta Otolaryngol* 1980;89:222–226.
44. Fell PJ, Soulsby S, Brostoff J. Cellular responses to food in irritable bowel syndrome—an investigation of the ALCAT test. *J Nutritional Med* 1991;2:143–149.
45. Donovan PN. The Elisa ACT test: its role in identifying time-delayed reactive environmental toxicants. *Townsend Letter for Doctors* 1991;5:???
46. Nolte H. Histamine release in food. *Hypersensitivity, Immunol Allergy Pract* 1991;12:10.
47. Sampson HA, et al. Spontaneous release of histamine from basophils and histamine releasing factor. *N Engl J Med* 1989;321:228–232.

Appendix 5–1

Dixon's Modified Directions for the Use of Vivonex or Tolorex

1. Place one package of Vivonex (300 cal.) in a blender or food processor.
2. Add one flavor package (orange-pineapple or lemon-lime are the most acceptable flavors to most patients).
3. Add 10–12 oz. (a tall glass) of water and mix for 4–5 minutes.
4. Pour about two thirds of the mixture into another container and refrigerate temporarily.
5. To the one third mixture remaining, add 3–4 ice cubes and crush in the blender or food processor, making it the consistency of a "slushy."
6. Sip this very slowly over a period of 25–30 minutes or longer.
7. Repeat with the next one third mixture. Take at *least* one hour to consume that complete package of mixture.

Some Notes

1. If you have one available, use a glass with a top and sip Vivonex through a straw. The odor is sometimes a problem, and a top keeps the odor to a minimum.
2. Always drink it very cold—this enhances taste and reduces the odor.
3. You must use at least five whole packages per day (1500 cal.) and, if the doctor prescribes, six.
4. Drink 4–6 large glasses of water every day you are on Vivonex.
5. If you are using Vivonex at work and do not have a blender available to crush ice, place a whole mixed package in a thermos without ice. Pour it over ice cubes as you need it, using only one third to one quarter of the mixture at a time.
6. Vivonex contains no food antigens and yet is complete nutrition if you take in 1500–2000 calories a day.
7. Vivonex is particularly useful in food allergy patients, both as a diagnostic test (together with total food and drink abstinence) and for periodic control of food symptoms.

8. A full two-week period on Vironex is necessary to clear all food antigens from the system in order to use this as a diagnostic test or as a means of controlling symptoms.

Appendix 5–2

Instructions for Preparing Test Meals for Challenge Food Test

Test Meals

1. *Wheat*—2 servings of Cream of Wheat, Wheatena or Ralston cooked in spring water and a little salt. Bring to test in thermos. Can also use puffed wheat or shredded wheat.
2. *Corn*—2 servings of corn meal mush, lightly salted. Bring in thermos. Also use corn popped in corn oil, or grits, or fresh corn on or off the cob.
3. *Egg*—3 hard or soft boiled eggs.
4. *Milk*—1 quart, in glass container if possible.
5. *Orange*—2 medium, whole.
6. *Potato*—2 large baked potatoes. Do not grease potatoes before baking.
7. *Beef*—3 slices roast or home ground round steak, broiled. May be lightly salted, not peppered or otherwise seasoned.
8. *Pork*—Same as beef. Cured ham is not pork. It is pork and several other products.
9. *Chicken*—2 servings, stewed or baked. No additional seasonings.
10. *Sugar*—2 tablespoons in glass of spring water. Stir well. May use sugar cubes.
11. *Coffee*—2 cups, black, made from patient's brand.
12. *Tea*—same as coffee.
13. *Chocolate*—eat Baker's chocolate or grate 3-one ounce squares in cold spring water.
14. *Other fruits*—fresh if possible (peeled), also water packed or dried stewed.
15. *Other vegetables*—same as other fruit.
16. *Baker's yeast*—one package additive free yeast from health food store in glass of ice cold spring water.
17. *Brewer's yeast*—found in health food store. Mix one tablespoon in glass of cold spring water.
18. *Food coloring*—use set of French's or McCormick's food colors. Mix together 1/2 teaspoon each color. Put 1 teaspoon of mixture in glass of spring water, drink.
19. *Soy*—tofu fried in Crisco, or margarine on rice cracker.

20. *Legumes*—2 servings of beans, black-eyed peas or beans of your choice.
21. *Peanuts*—dry roasted, unsalted peanuts or peanut butter from health food store. (no sugar, salt or preservatives.)

Source of errors: Errors in testing may be due to failure in complying with these instructions. *Read label carefully.* Prepare foods without additional ingredients.

Avoid starting test if increase in symptoms are present. Test may be delayed until day 6, 7, or 8 if necessary.

Appendix 5-3

Intradermal Provocative Food Test Form

(Example)

Patient: _John Doe_

Date: _____

Allergen Tested: _Corn_

Sx Relevant to Test: _Migraine Headaches_

Time Line in Minutes

	0	10	20	30	40	50	60	70	80	90	100	110	120	130
Glycerine Control	.05/1													
Wheal Size	9mm	11mm	11mm	9mm										
1st Test Dose	.05/1													
Wheal Size	9mm	13mm	13mm	13mm	11mm	9mm								
2nd Test Dose		.05/2												
Wheal Size		9mm	11mm	11mm	11mm	9mm	0							
3rd Test Dose				.05/3										
Wheal Size				9mm	9mm	9mm	0							
4th Test Dose														
Wheal Size					9mm	9mm	9mm	0						

	0	10	20	30	40	50
Signs	None	None Rhino-rrhea	Rhino-rrhea cough	Rhino-rrhea cough	Rhino-rrhea	None
Symptoms	None	Runny Nose	Runny Nose Cough	Runny Nose Cough	Runny Nose	None
Allergen injection	Corn	Corn		Corn		

Key:

.05/1 = 0.05cc of #1 dilution (1:100)

.05/2 = 0.05cc of #2 dilution (1:500)

.05/3 = 0.05cc of #3 dilution (1:2500)

Test:

Positive [ ]

Negative [X]

Neutralizing Dose #3 dilution (1:2500)

◆ 6 ◆

Nutrition Management in Food Allergy

Lynn Danford, M.S., and Manisha H. Maskay, Ph.D.

Human nutrition is a complex process that is critical to survival and health. The presence of food allergies can often compromise an individual's nutritional status. Malnutrition is associated with increased morbidity and poorer treatment outcomes. Attention to adequate nutrition must be an essential component of food allergy treatment.

Appropriate nutrition management can:

1. Promote nutritional adequacy and contribute to improved health
2. Enhance outcome of food allergy treatment
3. Improve management of comorbid conditions
4. Foster a sense of well being

To provide appropriate nutrition care, health care practitioners must have adequate knowledge of the principles of human nutrition, the components of a healthy diet, and the complexities of dietary behavior. In treating food allergies, it is also necessary to be knowledgeable about food sources of nutrients, botanical relationships, food composition, cooking methods, and alternative products and where they are available. Dietary modifications typically involve changes in lifestyle and are usually not easily accomplished. Clinicians with counseling skills as well as patience and sensitivity will be better able to assist individuals in complying with recommendations and achieving the desired results.

Enabling patients to accomplish dietary change is a sequential process that requires time and careful consideration of expected outcome versus cost to the patient. A complete assessment, the development and implementation of a realistic plan, ongoing follow-up, and evaluation are essential to improving outcome. Professional nutrition specialists are uniquely qualified to provide assistance in this area. If services of a nutrition specialist are not available, physicians and nurses involved in treating food allergy must receive adequate training in both the science and art of nutrition.

This chapter will explain how nutrition care can contribute to the treatment of patients with food allergy.

Role of Nutrition

Basics of Human Nutrition

Good nutrition provides the fundamental basis for health. Six categories of essential nutrients are required by the body for growth and normal functioning: carbohydrates, proteins, fats, vitamins, minerals, and water. The macronutrients—carbohydrates, proteins, and fats—supply energy and are required in large amounts. Vitamins and minerals, the micronutrients, are required in relatively small amounts.

Recommended Dietary Allowances (RDAs)

The Food and Nutrition Board of the National Academy of Sciences has established Recommended Dietary Allowances[1] which are defined as the levels of intake of essential nutrients that, on the basis of scientific knowledge, are judged to meet the known nutrient needs of practically all healthy persons. The estimated safe and adequate daily dietary intakes (ESADDI) are established for those nutrients for which the database is incomplete (see Appendix 6–1). The levels in both cases are those that prevent deficiencies and meet basic physiological requirements for normal, healthy individuals. These are not necessarily optimal amounts, nor do they reflect special nutritional requirements arising from injury or disease.

Energy

To maintain physiological functions, a constant supply of energy is necessary. The principal dietary sources of energy are carbohydrates, proteins, and fats. Energy expenditure is determined by age, gender, height, weight, activity level, and needs for growth, and therefore energy requirements must be calculated an individual basis.

Carbohydrate

Carbohydrates may be categorized as sugars (mono- and disaccharides) and complex carbohydrates (polysaccharides). Dietary fibers are mostly indigestible complex carbohydrates. The main dietary complex carbohydrate is starch.

The primary function of carbohydrate is to supply energy. Inadequate intake of carbohydrate has several potential metabolic consequences. Fats can be used to meet energy needs, but in the absence of carbohydrates this process may result in an accumulation of ketones, electrolyte imbalance, and dehydration. Similarly, proteins can be converted to energy at the expense of other essential functions.

About 55 to 60% of the body's daily energy requirement should be supplied by carbohydrates, and most of these should be complex. Grains, cereals, legumes, vegetables, fruits, and milk are sources of carbohydrate. Except for milk, these foods are also often good sources of fiber. Adequate dietary fiber is important and adults should consume approximately 20 to 35 grams per day; intakes that are significantly higher are not recommended.

Protein

Proteins are composed of amino acids, which are the fundamental structural components of cells. Eight amino acids are considered dietary essentials because they are not synthesized by humans. Plant proteins are considered incomplete because they do not contain sufficient amounts of the essential amino acids, and individuals who rely on plant proteins must pay special attention to obtaining an adequate intake of these amino acids.

Proteins are critical for growth and development. Protein can also supply energy through the process of gluconeogenesis. About 10 to 15% of the body's daily energy requirement should be supplied by protein. Animal sources of protein—including meat, poultry, seafood, egg, and milk—provide all the essential amino acids. Plant sources such as grains, cereals, soy products, legumes, nuts, and seeds may lack one or more essential amino acid.

Fat

Dietary fats are primarily triglycerides, which are composed of saturated fatty acids (SFA), monounsaturated fatty acids (MUFA), and polyunsaturated fatty acids (PUFA). Dietary fat is a concentrated source of energy and is required to transport fat-soluble vitamins and to supply essential fatty acids (EFA). EFAs are structural components of cell membranes and are precursors of prostaglandins, thromboxanes, leukotrienes, and certain hormones. Two additional roles of fat in the diet are to enhance satiety and palatability.

Fat should supply no more than 30% of daily energy requirements, with SFA, MUFA, and PUFA each contributing approximately 10%. Although excessive dietary fat is related to the development of many health problems, fat must not be excluded from the diet. Food sources of fat include animal and plant products. It is the primary component of many spreads, salad dressing, vegetable oils, and cream and is also found in baked products, meats, poultry, nuts, olives, and some milk products.

Vitamins

Vitamins are organic substances that, in general, cannot be produced in adequate amounts by the human body and are therefore dietary essentials. Vitamins are categorized as fat and water-soluble. Vitamins A, D, E, and K dissolve in organic solvents and thus fall in the fat-soluble category; the B vitamins and vitamin C are water-soluble.

Vitamins are required by the body in trace amounts to support normal functioning, growth, and maintenance of body tissues. They do not produce energy, but some vitamins are part of energy-producing chemical reactions. If the diet is lacking in a vitamin for an extended period of time, a deficiency state will develop that may eventually result in serious symptoms. Conversely, some vitamins, if consumed in megadoses, will over time result in toxicity.

Both plant and animal foods provide vitamins. A balanced diet that includes sufficient quantities of food from the various major food groups is most likely to ensure adequate vitamin intake.

Minerals

Minerals are inorganic substances that are categorized according to how much is required daily. Those required in amounts greater than 100 mg are referred to as major minerals; trace minerals are required in smaller amounts. Minerals are required for many, diverse metabolic roles and are critical to maintaining body function because of their involvement at the cellular, tissue, organ, and whole organism level.

A diet deficient in one more minerals will eventually result in serious deficiency symptoms. Excessive intake of minerals can also easily cause toxicity. If mineral supplements are recommended because of dietary deficiency, amounts greater than the RDA should be used with caution.

Water

Water plays several key roles in biological processes and is a major constituent of the human body. Regular intake is essential in order to compensate for daily losses because water is not conserved by the body to a sufficient degree.

Nutrition Assessment

A comprehensive nutrition assessment that includes a consideration of anthropometric, biochemical, clinical, dietary, and social parameters should be incorporated into the management of patients with food allergy. Careful evaluation of these factors provides the basis for nutrition recommendations and will contribute to successful outcomes.

Patient History

PAST AND PRESENT HISTORY OF ALLERGY SYMPTOMS AND REACTIONS

This includes anything the patient can recall as well as documentation of anaphylactic episodes from the medical record. Patients should be asked to described their perceptions about allergy symptoms, causes, frequency and severity. Details about season, location, and environmental factors are also relevant. Additionally, it is necessary to assess how seriously the individual's lifestyle is affected by the allergy.

WEIGHT AND WEIGHT HISTORY

Weight is a major indicator of health status. Dietary changes recommended in management of food allergy can contribute to changes in body weight which may be beneficial or detrimental.

Patients should be weighed at each visit and any changes in weight evaluated.

PSYCHOSOCIAL HISTORY

Many lifestyle factors can affect a patient's ability and willingness to implement dietary changes. A thorough evaluation and understanding of these factors provides vital data on which to base individual nutrition recommendations.

Economic status. Income level affects the amount of money available to purchase foods and to eat out. This is an influential factor if a patient must purchase special foods.

Occupation. Occupation influences daily schedule by determining when and perhaps where meals are consumed.

Educational background. Reading skills affect how well patients can comprehend written materials and instructions. Additionally, the ability to determine the content of individual foods from food labels can affect compliance with allergy diets.

Living situation. The presence of others in a household can influence the ability of one family member to implement changes. Persons responsible for food preparation may not be enthusiastic about the additional time and effort involved in preparing separate meals.

Stress level. The presence of excessive stressors can be a barrier to any type of dietary or lifestyle change. The degree of stress in a patient's life should be assessed so that the care plan is reasonable and does not present an additional source of stress.

Cultural norms. Dietary patterns are often related to religious and ethnic influences that are a part of each person's background.

Alcohol or tobacco use. The use of both substances can affect an individual's lifestyle, allergy symptoms, and nutritional status.

MEDICAL HISTORY

It is important to review the patient's medical history to determine the presence of additional health problems and to assess potential effects of dietary recommendations. A brief review should include but not be limited to:

- Gastrointestinal concerns such as gastroesophageal reflux, irritable bowel syndrome, inflammatory bowel disease, constipation, diarrhea, vomiting, or general discomfort
- Hyperlipidemia
- Diabetes mellitus
- Anemia
- Eating disorders (anorexia nervosa and bulimia nervosa) *The presence or suspicion of anorexia nervosa should be of particular concern to clinicians. Elimination diets used in the treatment of food allergy can exacerbate this condition.*

The use of prescription and nonprescription medications should also be reviewed.

The use of any nutritional supplements should be determined. It is not enough to learn that a patient takes "vitamins." The exact content and dose should be ascertained. Supplements can contain substances with allergenic potential. Patients should be instructed to bring products into the office for evaluation.

DIET HISTORY

A thorough diet history is necessary. Knowledge of typical eating patterns will enable the clinician to evaluate nutrition adequacy and to more successfully adapt nutrition recommendations to the patient's lifestyle. Factors to consider are:

- Food preferences, including foods avoided
- Number of meals eaten each day
- Typical meals, beverages, and snacks
- Frequency of meals prepared at home and meals eaten out
- Special dietary considerations (eg, vegetarian, low fat, kosher)

Clinical and Biochemical Indicators

Weight is an important indicator of health status. Patients with weights notably higher or lower than normal are at increased risk for various health problems. The body mass index (BMI) is a well-accepted indicator of appropriate weight for height (Table 6–1).

Rapid loss of weight, or weight notably different from the patient's usual weight can also be critical indicators of nutritional status (Table 6–2).

Promotion of Nutritional Adequacy

A fundamental understanding of basic nutrition requirements and a concern for maintaining optimal nutrition status are imperative. Dietary interventions should be carefully planned so that patients with food allergy continue to consume adequate amounts of energy and all essential nutrients. In addition, the inclusion of the greatest variety of food substances possible should be encouraged. Diagnostic and therapeutic programs that omit sources of vital

Table 6–1   Using BMI for Assessing Weight

BMI	$BMI = \dfrac{weight\ (kilograms)}{height^2\ (meters)}$
<20	Below normal weight for height
20–25	Normal weight for height
25–30	Overweight
>30	Obese

Table 6–2   Checklist for Assessing Nutritional Status

- ☐ BMI <20 or >30.
- ☐ Rapid weight loss (≥5% of body weight in 1 month)
- ☐ Major weight loss (≥10% in 6 months)
- ☐ Low serum albumin (<3.5 g/dL)
- ☐ Low serum cholesterol (<130 mg/dL)
- ☐ Poor appetite

Positive response to any of the above may indicate increased risk for compromised nutritional status.

nutrients without adequate substitutes can cause malnutrition and result in further health problems.

The Food Guide pyramid (Fig. 6–1) is a useful guideline for both clinicians and patients. It can be used to promote appropriate food selection from the key food categories and thus optimize nutritional status.

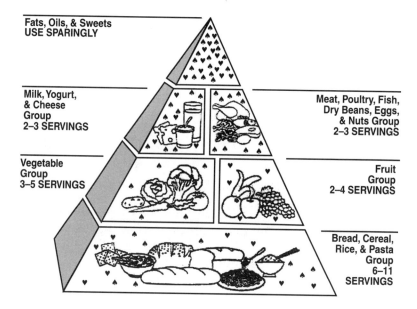

Serving sizes:

Bread/Cereal/Rice/Pasta	Bread	1 slice
	Ready-to-eat cereal	1 oz
	Cooked cereal/rice pasta	$^1/_2$ cup
	Plain creakers	3–4
Vegetables/Fruits	Raw	1 cup
	Cooked	$^1/_2$ cup
	Juice	$^3/_4$ cup
	Apple, banana, orange, etc.	1 medium
Milk/Yogurt/Cheese	Milk/yogurt	1 cup
	Cheese	1 $^1/_2$ oz
Meat/Poultry/Fish/Eggs/	Cooked meat/poultry/fish	2–3 oz
Dried beans/Nuts	Cooked beans	$^1/_2$ cup
	Egg	1 = 1 oz meat
	Peanut butter	2 tbsp. = 1 oz meat

Figure 6–1. The Food Guide Pyramid—A Guide to Daily Food Choices. ♠ Fat (naturally occuring and added); ♥ Sugars (added). These symbols show fat and added sugars in foods. Source: U.S. Department of Agriculture.

Diagnostic Procedures

Appropriate procedures are necessary to accurately diagnose food allergy and to identify the specific food triggers. When there is a history of immediate and life-threatening reactions to a specific food, diagnostic protocols are typically superfluous. The context of the situation, including the immediacy and severity of the reaction, provides adequate identification of the offending food. However, when reactions are delayed, symptoms are less severe, or there is a lack of information about food composition, it can be more difficult to identify the allergens.

Inaccurate diagnoses or overdiagnoses of food allergies must be avoided. Symptoms incorrectly attributed to food allergy may prevent recognition of another disorder. For example, gastrointestinal conditions such as lactose intolerance and gluten enteropathy may be confused with food allergy. In addition, dietary restrictions used in elimination diets can cause nutrient deficiencies that may lead to various clinical symptoms. Finally, patients who have been incorrectly diagnosed may develop a fear of food, which can create lifelong difficulties with eating.

Diagnostic procedures include several steps: the history, food and symptom diary, elimination trial, and oral food challenges. A careful evaluation of these components is essential for identifying food allergies, developing a treatment plan, and determining the results of the treatment.

Evaluation of Diet History

The diet history may reveal that the patient avoids certain foods. The reasons for eliminating foods should be ascertained. Individuals may instinctively omit foods because of a food sensitivity, without actually identifying it as such.

Foods may be omitted for other reasons, including misconceptions about food sensitivities. Confusion about the association between foods and allergy symptoms abounds; thus, people may incorrectly believe that a particular food causes symptoms.

Food and Symptom Diary

Careful patient self-monitoring and record keeping provide data that is critical for diagnosing food allergies (Table 6–3). Although journal keeping is a time-consuming endeavor, both clinicians and patients will recognize the value. Most important, this record establishes a baseline for symptoms and complaints. Second, it can help identify suspected food allergens and assess the severity of reactions, dose-dependant relationships, and the role of cooking in making foods more tolerable. Finally, not only does a diary help detect reactions to foods, it can be extremely useful in ruling them out.

Table 6–3   Food and Symptom Diary Instructions for Patients

Instructions for keeping your daily food and symptom diary:

1. Record all foods, beverages, snacks, supplements, and medicines of any type.

2. List ingredients of combination foods such as casseroles, stews, and salads.

3. Record all symptoms and indicate when they started. Indicate the severity by using a scale of 1 to 4.

4. Complete the diary as the day progresses; do not wait until the end of the week as it is too difficult to remember what happened.

5. Complete a diary each day until your next appointment.

6. Bring all information to your next appointment.

Sample Diet Diary

TIME	FOOD EATEN	TIME	SYMPTOMS/ SEVERITY SCALE
8:00	banana 1 boiled egg 1 cup orange juice 1 piece toast/butter	8:15	throat itching—2
10:15	1 cup grapes	10:18	lips swelling—1
12:30	hot dog, bun	1:00	no symtoms

Providing adequate verbal and written instructions to patients will facilitate accurate record keeping. The food diary should be maintained for at least 10 to 14 days. The information will require scrupulous evaluation at the following clinic visit. It may be possible to infer relationships between food and symptoms based on the chronology.

Elimination Trial

Careful review of the allergy tests, the diet history, and the food and symptom diary will usually suggest which foods may be triggering symptoms. An elimination diet can then be utilized to *identify* suspected foods and substantiate cause-and-effect relationships. Permanent dietary restrictions are not instituted at this point.

Some clinicians prefer to use a rotary and elimination diet. This requires more involved instruction because the patient is allowed to consume only certain foods each day. Patients should be encouraged to avoid eating the same foods every day.

Adequate instructions and resources are essential for patients who are beginning elimination diets. Individuals cannot realistically be expected to change lifelong food patterns without sufficient information and support. The following steps are useful:

- State which foods, types of food, and combination dishes are to be omitted. Review the patient's food diary and specify sources of the food in question.
- List which foods may be eaten and emphasize the variety and scope. Note that the same foods should not be eaten every day.
- Discuss substitutes for foods commonly eaten, as reported in the food diary. This can be done meal by meal (ie, breakfast, lunch and dinner choices). Alternatively, suggestions can be made by food group (eg, protein-containing foods, fruits, vegetables). The food pyramid (Fig. 6) is helpful.
- Provide suggestions for beverages and snacks.
- Encourage consumption of as great a variety of foods as possible.
- Supply instructions on how to read and evaluate labels, including how to recognize the various terms which are used to describe ingredients (Table 6–4).
- Discuss where alternative foods, when necessary, can be obtained. Supermarkets in large metropolitan areas now carry a wide range of food products. Other good sources are health food stores, ethnic groceries, and mail order suppliers (Appendix 6–2).
- Define a specific period of time for the plan to be followed. Two weeks is a reasonable minimum. The patient should continue to keep food and symptom diaries while following the elimination diet.
- Have available additional information such as recipes, product information (Appendix 6–3), and cookbook references (Appendix 6–4).
- Instruct patients to report any nonfood contributors to symptoms such as environmental exposures.

A follow-up visit or telephone contact after about 2 weeks of an elimination diet is beneficial to both the clinician and the patient. It enables the clinician to assess compliance and identify problems. If the care plan has not been correctly implemented, it is necessary to determine the reasons. Often further instructions, such as specific meal planning guidelines, are required. Family conflicts, financial limitations, or a lack of motivation, among other factors, can also be barriers to compliance. These types of problems should be addressed in a sensitive and instructive way (see Strategies to Promote Dietary Change).

Optimally, having followed the elimination plan for 2 or more weeks, the patient will return with an improvement in allergy manifestations. The log will verify that the instructions have been followed and the foods in question

Table 6–4   Names for Sources of Common Allergens

Wheat:	graham flour, cereal extract, whole wheat, bran
Milk:	casein, caseinate, dry milk solids, whey
Egg:	albumin, ovo-mucin, ovoglobulin
Corn:	dextrose, corn syrup, corn starch

have been eliminated. The documented symptoms, when compared to baseline, will also provide information regarding progress in frequency, severity, and/or duration of symptoms.

The follow-up visit should include an assessment of:

• Nutritional status
• Symptoms
• Change in symptoms from baseline
• Compliance with guidelines
• Problems experienced

A decision can be made to continue the elimination program; begin oral food challenges, which are the next phase in the diagnostic procedure; or discontinue the elimination trial.

If there is no evidence of improvement, it may be that (1) not enough time has elapsed; (2) the foods being tested were not entirely omitted; (3) the identification of the offending foods was inaccurate; or (4) the diagnosis of food allergy can be ruled out.

Food and symptom logs should be carefully reviewed to determine if the elimination diet guidelines were correctly followed, and if any exacerbations occurred. Food and nonfood precipitants may be involved. Reliable evidence of an additional food allergen is documentation that every time the food was ingested in the same form (ie, raw or cooked), symptoms resulted.

Oral Food Challenges

Oral food challenges (OFC) help confirm the diagnosis of food allergy and assess the severity of the condition. They are best initiated when the prescribed diet has been followed for at least 5 days, the symptoms are stabilized, and the patient is in good general health.

A single-blinded, placebo-controlled challenge performed in the clinic office is the gold standard method, but a procedure that patients can follow at home, using ordinary foods, is also useful. The instructions below (Table 6–5) outline a protocol that is relatively easy for patients to follow. This method will provide relevant information to both the clinician and the patient about the relationship between food and symptoms. If a reaction occurs and the patient perceives the cause-and-effect relationship between food and symptoms, it reinforces a belief in the diagnosis and the consequences of food allergy. The presence of this belief is critical to successful treatment.

Challenges are obviously contraindicated in any patient with severe, life-threatening food allergy.

Challenges should be completed for one food at a time. The suggestions in Table 6–6 provide suitable choices.

It is important that outcomes of the OFC are carefully reviewed after completion of the protocol so that the presence of food allergies is either

Table 6–5 Patient Instructions for Oral Food Challenges

IF SYMPTOMS OCCUR AT ANY TIME DURING THIS PROCEDURE, THE TEST IS POSITIVE. OMIT THE FOOD AND DO NOT PROCEED FURTHER. CONTACT YOUR HEALTH CARE PRACTITIONER.

The foods to be challenged are _____, _____, _____ .

Challenge one food at a time and complete all the steps before proceeding to the next food. Continue keeping a dairy throughout the food challenge procedure. Your complete involvement is essential in this process.

1. Include the suspected food in the diet daily for 4 days.

2. Omit the suspected food and all products made with it for the following 4 days. Do not be concerned if you do not become symptom-free.

3. On the next day (food testing day), eat a normal breakfast omitting the food to be tested. Do not perform the test this day if ill, or if allergy symptoms are more severe than usual. The challenge procedure may be postponed.

4. Three to 4 hours after breakfast, eat a large, typical serving of the suspected food with nothing added except water. Observe any symptoms for 1 hour. During this time provide a comfortable environment and avoid exposure to any other substances that might produce confusing allergic symptoms.

5. At the end of the first hour, if no signs or symptoms occur, eat a second portion of the food. Watch for symptoms for the next 30 to 60 minutes.

6. Eat lunch without the suspected food.

7. Include the suspected food again at the evening meal.

8. Watch for delayed onset of symptoms during the next 24 hours.

9. If a positive test is obtained, do not eat the food or any of its products until the results are discussed with your health care practitioner.

Outcomes of the food challenges may be meaningful to the ongoing management of your allergies. Please be sure to inform your health care practitioner of both positive and negative results.

---

substantiated or ruled out. Both the patient's impressions and the documentation provided in the food diaries are useful for making the diagnosis.

Patients themselves are usually able to recognize if reactions were provoked. In the case of a positive test, the patient's involvement in the diagnostic process fosters an understanding of the relationship between ingestion of certain foods and symptoms, thus strengthening the belief in the existence of a food allergy. Alternatively, the absence of any symptoms from the food provocation effectively eliminates the diagnosis of food allergy.

Without this final procedure of evaluating the results of OFC, uncertainty about the diagnosis will persist. It is in the best interest of both the clinician and the patient to have this information available for planning treatment.

Table 6–6   Recommended Foods for Challenges

Wheat:	cream of wheat cereal, pasta, bulgur wheat, couscous, matzo crackers, any other bread or crakers made without yeast, milk, egg, etc.
Corn:	corn on the cob, canned or frozen corn, popcorn, corn meal
Milk:	milk, plain yogurt
Soy:	soy milk, tofu, soy nuts
Orange:	fresh orange, orange juice
Egg:	boiled or poached egg
Peanut:	peanuts or peanut butter
Yeast:	bread (if no evidence of wheat allergy), baker's yeast powder stirred in water or juice, rye or other wheat-free crackers containing yeast

Treatment

When to Treat—Costs vs. Benefits

As with any type of medical intervention, a decision to treat is based on the evidence available and on weighing costs versus benefits. The patient's well-being depends on many factors. Clearly food allergies present a health risk. Depending on the severity of the symptoms and reactions, however, the benefits of treating the condition with dietary restrictions may be outweighed by the costs. Health care providers who recommend dietary changes should be sensitive to the difficulty of such an endeavor. Exacting dietary modifications can require profound lifestyle changes, representing psychological, social, and practical sacrifices to the patient.

In addition, there are strong medical contraindications to using an elimination diet as treatment. These conditions are not always obvious and include (1) excessive weight loss, (2) undernutrition, and (3) anorexia nervosa. Clinicians will be more likely to detect the existence of these potentially serious problems by taking a complete history and following the patients' progress during the diagnostic phase.

Weight loss will be detected if patients' weights are checked and documented during each office visit. In addition, any weight change that is unacceptable to the patient, even if specific criteria are not met, should not be ignored. Loss of body mass can represent a serious health risk, especially in the elderly.

The risk of inappropriate weight loss and malnutrition can increase as a result of an elimination diet for several reasons. The most common cause is a lack of skills or knowledge necessary to prepare alternative foods. Patients may subsist on a meager diet, resulting in inadequate energy and nutrient intake. Additionally, loss of appetite and lack of enjoyment of eating can occur with the elimination of favorite foods from the diet. In other cases, the effort required to change food consumption patterns is just too extensive; patients may feel it is ultimately easier to forgo eating in order to avoid the difficulties.

Any evidence of an eating disorder should be taken very seriously. Anorexia nervosa is a dangerous condition characterized by severe, self-imposed dietary restrictions. An elimination diet used in the treatment of food allergy encourages the omission of additional foods from the diet, making it even more difficult for patients to maintain adequate energy and nutrient intake.

Weighing risks and benefits in developing treatment strategies should take into account both the type and severity of the condition. Not all food sensitivities are food allergies, nor do they all represent a risk to the patient. For example, a sensitivity to milk (lactose intolerance) can generally be treated without the elimination of milk products.

Assessing the severity of the condition requires not only the clinical evaluation of symptoms but also the patient's perceptions of how critically his or her lifestyle is affected. The extent to which a person's health and well-being is affected by the allergy will influence treatment planning. If the symptoms are mild and tolerable to the patient, the food allergy may not be serious enough to justify the effort required for treatment with dietary modification. Patients should be involved in deciding treatment strategies. Some individuals will prefer to tolerate mild manifestations. Others will welcome dietary manipulations as the optimal treatment for controlling troublesome symptoms. Still others will resist dietary strategies and prefer to use available pharmacological agents if possible.

Strategies to Promote Dietary Change

There are potentially many obstacles to changing dietary patterns. Identification of the practical and emotional barriers that prevent compliance can help clinicians effectively address issues and problems.

If patients acknowledge that family conflicts about food and eating are a problem, it is helpful to emphasize the types of food that can be eaten by everyone—for example, meat, potatoes, vegetables, and fruits. Sauces, dressings, and gravies can be served on the side. Financial concerns may be perceived rather than genuine. Food dollars can often be saved with the omission of snack foods, prepared foods, and purchased beverages. Simply prepared protein-containing foods, vegetables, and starches such as rice or potatoes are not as costly as other frequently consumed food products.

Managing a lack of motivation can be more challenging. Numerous studies in behavioral psychology and medicine have investigated what factors motivate changes in health-related behaviors. The Health Belief Model[2] describes the importance of predisposing enabling and reinforcing factors in promoting behavior change. The presence of negative beliefs or the lack of enabling and reinforcing factors may hinder behavioral change. Conversely, the presence of positive beliefs will foster behavior change. These include:

1. A belief in personal susceptibility to a disease
2. A belief that the disease presents a threat to health and well-being
3. A belief that the recommended health action will be effective in reducing the threat or severity of the condition
4. A belief that the barriers associated with following health recommendations are outweighed by benefits
5. A belief in self-efficacy to carry out instructions

If one or more of these beliefs is absent, it can hamper implementation of the care plan. Clinicians who address barriers to behavior change and foster a sense of self-efficacy will have more success getting patients to follow dietary recommendations. For example, the belief in susceptibility may be absent because of the lack of recognition of a relationship between allergy symptoms and diet. Delayed or subtle reactions to commonly consumed foods are not easily identified, and therefore individuals deny the existence of food allergy and its impact on health. This belief can be developed by providing information and enhancing understanding about food allergy mechanisms. Also, involving patients in the review of food and symptom logs can enhance recognition of the role of foods in exacerbating symptoms. The involved patient is more likely to appreciate the impact of food allergy on health.

Elimination Diet

Extensive instructions are imperative for patients requiring long-term dietary modifications if compliance with the program and control of symptoms are to be accomplished successfully. Guidelines must assure avoidance of allergens and promote overall health and well-being by following sound nutritional principles and minimizing costs to the patient.

The following checklist (Table 6–7) is useful for planning elimination diets with patients. A list of alternate foods follows (Table 6–8).

Suggested places to shop for such foods include supermarkets, ethnic groceries (Chinese, Japanese, Indian), health food stores, and mail order suppliers. A large amount of information about food choices, meal planning, and the management of food allergies is also available through books, pamphlets, manufacturers, and on computer networks (see Appendices 6-2 to 6-5). Resourceful patients who take advantage of these materials will find both helpful information and support in their efforts.

Long-term management of patients with food allergies who are following elimination diets should include a periodic review of symptoms and ongoing assessment of nutritional status.

Table 6–7   Patient Guidelines for Maintaining a Nutritionally Balanced Elimination Diet

The foods to be avoided are: _____

The foods that can be eaten are: _____

Concentrate first on the foods that can be eaten, rather than on those that must be avoided.

Include sources of the basic nutrients by eating according to the Food Pyramid.

Substitutes for favorite foods at breakfast, lunch, and dinner include: _____

Substitutes for favorite beverages include: _____

Concentrate on the basics and keep meals simple. Meats, poultry, fish, vegetables, potato, rice, salads, and fruit provide excellent choices. Serve or request dressings and sauces on the side.

Try new foods for more variety.

Be open minded—forego traditions for breakfast, lunch, and dinner foods if desired.

Always read and evaluate food labels carefully.

Make or buy large quantities of appropriate foods. Eat leftovers and/or freeze extras.

Plan ahead for dining out and special occasions.

Ask questions about food content and preparation techniques when dining out.

Dealing with Associated Health Problems

Attention should be paid to the impact of any allergy diet on comorbid conditions such as excessive weight loss, anorexia nervosa, obesity, diabetes,

Table 6–8   Alternative Foods Useful in an Elimination Diet (see Appendix 6–2 for resource information)

Many suitable products are available commercially.

Milk substitutes:
Beverages made from nuts, rice, soy (calcium-fortified are preferred)

Starch substitutes:
Crackers made from rye, oat, rice
Pasta made from corn, buckwheat, rice
Cooked grains: barley, quinoa, millet, oat, buckwheat, rye, tapioca, rice, potato, wild rice, amaranth
Legumes
Bread made from rice, soy, millet
Spaghetti squash

Peanut substitutes:
Nuts, nut butters (almond, cashew, etc), sesame seeds, sesame butter (tahini)

or gastrointestinal disease. It is important to avoid confusing and contradictory recommendations. These situations call for highly skilled and specialized attention.

Conclusion

Nutrition is an essential component in the diagnosis and treatment of food allergy. Nutrition recommendations based on careful assessment will enhance treatment outcomes. The process of changing diet and eating behaviors is complicated and requires ongoing attention, commitment, knowledge, and self-efficacy. Health care practitioners who treat food allergy must provide patients with the information and skills to implement recommendations that are part of the diagnostic and treatment process.

The goal of nutrition care is to improve health status without diminishing the quality of life or compromising nutrition status. It should involve individualized guidance regarding food and nutrient intake, taking into account the individual's cultural, socioeconomic, health, functional, and psychological status. For food allergy patients, it may include counseling to decrease intake of certain nutrients or foods and increase intake of others. Recommendations should be based on careful assessment of cost versus benefit, taking into consideration not only the specific health problem but the whole person. Overly restrictive diets should be avoided as much as possible. The services of a nutrition specialist should be utilized to enable the patient to accomplish dietary change without excessive discomfort and to consume a balanced diet that provides pleasure and satisfaction in addition to improving health status.

Appendix 6–1

Recommended Daily Allowances[a]

		Weight[b]		Height[b]			Fat-Soluble Vitamins			
Category	Age (years) or Condition	(kg)	(lb)	(cm)	(in)	Protein (g)	Vita-min A (μg RE)[c]	Vita-min D (μg)[d]	Vita-min E (mg α-TE)[e]	Vita-min K (μg)
Infants	0.0–0.5	6	13	60	24	13	375	7.5	3	5
	0.5–1.0	9	20	71	28	14	375	10	4	10
Children	1–3	13	29	90	35	16	400	10	6	15
	4–6	20	44	112	44	24	500	10	7	20
	7–10	28	62	132	52	28	700	10	7	30
Males	11–14	45	99	157	62	45	1,000	10	10	10
	15–18	66	145	176	69	59	1,000	10	10	65
	19–24	72	160	177	70	58	1,000	10	10	70
	25–50	79	174	176	70	63	1,000	5	10	80
	51+	77	170	173	68	63	1,000	5	10	80
Females	11–14	46	101	157	62	46	800	10	8	45
	15–18	55	120	163	64	44	800	10	8	55
	19–24	58	128	164	65	46	800	10	8	60
	25–50	63	138	163	64	50	800	5	8	65
	51+	65	143	160	63	50	800	5	8	65
Pregnant						60	800	10	10	65
Lactating	1st 6 months					65	1,300	10	12	65
	2nd 6 months					62	1,200	10	11	65

[a] The allowances, expressed as average daily intakes over time, are intended to provide for individual variations among most normal persons as they live in the United States under usual environmental stresses. Diets should be based on a variety of common foods in order to provide other nutrients for which human requirements have been less well defined. See text for detailed discussion of allowances and of nutrients not tabulated.

[b] Weights and heights of Reference Adults are actual medians for the U.S. population of the designated age, as reported by NHANES II. The median weights and heights of those under 19 years of age were taken from Hamill et al. (1979) (see pages 16–17). The use of these figures does not imply that the height-to-weight rations are ideal.

[c] Retinol equivalents. 1 retinol equivalent = 1 μg retinol or 6 μg β-carotene. See text for calculation of vitamin A activity of diets as retinol equivalents.

[d] As cholecalciferol. 10 μg cholecalciferol = 400 IU of vitamin D.

[e] α-Tocopherol equivalents. 1 mg d-α tocopherol = 1 α-TE. See text for variation in allowances and calculation of vitamin E activity of the diet as α-tocopherol equivalents.

[f] 1 NE (niacin equivalent) is equal to 1 mg of niacin or 60 mg of dietary tryptophan.

Reprinted with permission from *Recommended Daily Allowances*, 10th ed. Copyright 1989 by the National Academy of Sciences. Courtesy of the National Academy of Sciences, Washington, D.C.

Water-Soluble Vitamins							Minerals						
Vitamin C (mg)	Thiamin (mg)	Riboflavin (mg)	Niacin (mg NE)^f	Vitamin B$_6$ (mg)	Folate (µg)	Vitamin B$_{12}$ (µg)	Calcium (mg)	Phosphorus (mg)	Magnesium (mg)	Iron (mg)	Zinc (mg)	Iodine (µg)	Selenium (µg)
30	0.3	0.4	5	0.3	25	0.3	400	300	40	6	5	40	10
35	0.4	0.5	6	0.6	35	0.5	600	500	60	10	5	50	15
40	0.7	0.8	9	1.0	50	0.7	800	800	80	10	10	70	20
45	0.9	1.1	12	1.1	75	1.0	800	800	120	10	10	90	20
50	1.3	1.5	17	1.7	150	2.0	1,200	1,200	270	12	15	150	40
60	1.5	1.8	20	2.0	200	2.0	1,200	1,200	400	12	15	150	50
60	1.5	1.7	19	2.0	200	2.0	1,200	1,200	350	10	15	150	70
60	1.5	1.7	19	2.0	200	2.0	800	800	350	10	15	150	70
60	1.2	1.4	15	2.0	200	2.0	800	800	350	10	15	150	70
50	1.1	1.3	15	1.4	150	2.0	1,200	1,200	280	15	12	150	45
60	1.1	1.3	15	1.5	180	2.0	1,200	1,200	300	15	12	150	50
60	1.1	1.3	15	1.6	180	2.0	1,200	1,200	280	15	12	150	55
60	1.1	1.3	15	1.6	180	2.0	800	800	280	15	12	150	55
60	1.0	1.2	13	1.6	180	2.0	800	800	280	10	12	150	55
70	1.5	1.6	17	2.2	400	2.2	1,200	1,200	320	30	15	175	65
95	1.6	1.8	20	2.1	280	2.6	1,200	1,200	355	15	19	200	75
90	1.6	1.7	20	2.1	260	2.6	1,200	1,200	340	15	16	200	75

Appendix 6–2

Resources for Alternative Foods

Ener-G Foods
P.O. Box 84487
Seattle, WA 98124–5787
800/331–5222
(extensive selection of products
including wheat-free bread,
pasta, cereals, crackers, cookies,
snacks, milk-free beverages, egg
replacer)

Modern Products, Inc.
P.O. Box 09398
Milwaukee, WI 53209
414/352–3209
(rice products)

Joyva Tahini
53 Varick Avenue
Brooklyn, NY 11237
718/497–0170
(sesame products)

Van's International Foods
Torrance CA 90501
(dairy-free frozen waffles, wheat-
free pancakes)

Arrowhead Mills
Box 2059
Hereford, TX 79045
(various grains, cereals; wheat-free
brownie mix)

Erewhon
U.S. Mills
Omaha, NE 68111
(grains, cereals)

Quaker Oats Co.
Chicago, IL 60654

Purity Foods Inc.
2871 W. Jolly Rd.
Okemos, MI 48864
517/351–9231
(grains)

Birkett Mills
P.O. Box 440
Penn Yan, NY 14527
(buckwheat products)

Rice Council of America
P.O. Box 740123
Houston, TX 77274
713/270–6699
(wild rice)

Quinoa Corp.
P.O. Box 1039
Torrance, CA 90505
(quinoa products)

Kölln NA
One Executive Drive
Fort Lee, NJ 07024
(cereals)

Barbara's Bakery
Petaluma, CA 94954
(cereals, snacks)

Health Valley
800/423–4846
(cereals)

New Morning
Acton, MA 01720
(cereals)

Nature's Path Foods, Inc.
Delta, BC V4G1E8
(oat cereal)

Lifestream Natural Foods
P.O. Box 8110
Blaine, WA 98230
(oat cereal)

Edward & Son Trading Co.
Box 1326
Carpenteria, CA 93014
(rice crackers)

Eden Foods
Clinton, MI
(grains, flours)

Westbrae
310/886–8200
(milk-free beverages)

Rice Dream
Imagine Foods
350 Cambridge Avenue #350
Palo Alto, CA 94306
(milk-free beverages)

Vita Soy Inc.
Brisbane, CA 94005
(milk-free beverages)

Amazake
Grainaissance Inc.
1580 62nd St.
Emeryville, CA 94608
(milk-free beverages)

Better than Milk?
Sovex Natural Foods
Box 2178
Collegedale, TN 37315
(milk-free beverages)

Solait
Devansoy Farms Inc.
P.O. Box 885
Carroll, IA 51401
800/747–8605
(milk-free beverages)

White Wave Inc.
Boulder, CO 80301
(milk-free beverages)

Wholesome & Hearty Foods
2422 SW Hawthorne Blvd.
Portland, OR 97214
800/636–0109
(almond milk)

Food for Life
2991 E. Doherty St.
Corona CA 91719
(rice & millet breads)
Tofutti Brands
Crawford NJ 07016
(milk-free ice cream)

Appendix 6–3

Alternative Foods

Flours and Grains:
amaranth
barley
buckwheat
corn
Jersulean artichoke
millet
oat
potato
quinoa
rice
rye
soy
tapioca

Ready-to-Eat Grain Products:
rye crackers
rye crispbread
rice cakes
corn cakes
rice noodles
buckwheat noodles
oat, rice, rye, buckwheat and millet cereals

Ready-to-Eat Snacks and Desserts:
soy ice cream
Italian ice
sorbet
potato chips
corn chips

Appendix 6–4

Cookbooks

The Allergy Cookie Jar. Carol Rudoff. Allergy Publications, 1985, 128 pp.
Allergy Gourmet: A Collection of Wheat-Free, Milk-Free, Egg-Free, Corn-Free, Soy-Free Recipes. Carol Rudoff. Allergy Publications, 1983, 225 pp.
Allergy Products Directory. Allergy Publications, 1987, 128 pp.
The Allergy Self-Help Cookbook. Marjore Hurt Jones. Rodale Press, 1984, 385 pp.
Cooking for People with Food Allergies. Human Nutrition Information Service. USDA Home and Garden Bulletin No. 246.
Coping With Food Allergy Claude A. Frazier. Random House, 1985, 325 pp.
Dairy Free Cookbook. Jane Zukin. Prima Publications and Communications, 1989, 300 pp.
Food Allergies. Merri Lou Dobler. The American Dietetic Association, 1991, 34 pp.
Food Allergy Cookbook. Allergy Information Association. St. Martin's Press, 1986, 137 pp.
The Gluten-Free Gourmet: Living Well Without Wheat. Betty Hagman. Holt, 1990, 256 pp.
Gluten Intolerance. Merri Lou Dobler. The American Dietetic Association, 1991, 25 pp.
Lactose Intolerance. Merri Lou Dobler. The American Dietetic Association, 1991, 21 pp.
The Milk Free Kitchen. Beth Kidden. Holt, 1991.
The Milk Sugar Dilemma: Living with Lactose Intolerance, 2nd ed. Richard A. Martens and Sherilyn Martens. Medi-Ed Press, 1987, 260 pp.
Wheat-Free Cooking. Ruby Brown. Sally Milner Publishing, 1990, 223 pp.
Wheatless Cooking. Ruth Shattuck. Signet, 1986, 319 pp.

Appendix 6–5

On-Line Information Sources

There is a large amount of information about food allegy available on the Internet. A few of these are listed.

Food Allergies
http://ww/sig/net/~allergy/food.html

The On-Line Allergy Center
http://www.sig.net/~allergy/welcome.html

The American Academy of Allergy, Asthma and Immunology
http://execpc.com/~edi/aaaai.html

The Allergy Shop
http://www.awod.com/gallerg/business/allergy/
http://www.pride-net.com/allergy/

Learning Resource Center
http://www/podi.com/health/aanma/aanlearn.html

Allergy and Asthma Web Page
http://www.cs.unc.edu/~kupstas/FAQ.html

Allergy Information Center
http://www.kww.com/allergy/

The Food Allergy Network
http://www.foodallergy.org/

References

1. National Research Council. *Recommended Dietary Allowances*, 10th ed. Washington, DC: National Academy Press, 1989.
2. Becker MH. The health belief model and personal health behavior. *Health Educ Monogr* 1974;2:324–508.

Index

Note: Figures and tables are represented by *f* and *t* respectively.